# Winning with Back Pain

**Other books from these authors:**

*Winning with Arthritis*

*Winning with Osteoporosis*

*The 50+ Wellness Program*

# Winning with Back Pain

Harris H. McIlwain, MD
Debra Fulghum Bruce
Joel C. Silverfield, MD
Michael C. Burnette, MD
Bernard F. Germain, MD

John Wiley & Sons, Inc.
New York • Chichester • Brisbane • Toronto • Singapore

This text is printed on acid-free paper.



***Library of Congress Cataloging in Publication Data:***

Winning with back pain / Harris H. McIlwain . . . [et al.].
p. cm.
Includes index.
ISBN 0-471-30328-3 (paper)
1. Backache—Treatment. 2. Backache—Prevention. I. McIlwain, Harris H.
RD771.B217W56 1994
617.5'64—dc20 93-8379

Printed in the United States of America

10 9 8 7 6 5 4 3 2 1

In memory of James Edward McIlwain, Sr.
Loyal husband, supportive father.
Loving grandfather, devoted friend.

# Contributors

We are grateful to the many talented professionals who contributed time and effort to make this book possible:

Francis I. Barford, L.O.T.R.

Dana S. Deboskey, Ph.D.

Arthur Frommer, Travel Editor

Roy E. Fulghum

Ann Hackney, R.N., B.S.N., M.A.

Susan Haley, R.D., L.D.

Dominador U. Martirez, R.P.T., L.P.T.

R. Wayne Miller, Esquire

Robert J. Rodriguez, D.C.

Rick Ruge, Supervisor, Media Services, University Community Hospital, Tampa, Florida

Stephen F. Russell, Ph.D.

Vernon L. Swenson, Ph.D.

Tampa Medical Group, P.A.

Vicki K. Windsor, R.P.T.

# Acknowledgments

We are grateful to the following for assisting in so many ways to get this book to press: Daniel, Ginah, Kimberly, Laura, Linda, and Michael McIlwain, and especially our editor, Judith McCarthy.

## TRADEMARKS

Advil is a trademark of Whitehall Laboratories, Inc.
Anacin 3 is a trademark of Whitehall Laboratories, Inc.
Anaprox is a trademark of Syntex Laboratories, Inc.
Anexsia is a trademark of Beecham Laboratories.
Ansaid is a trademark of The Upjohn Company.
Arthritis Strength Ascriptin is a trademark of Rorer Consumer Pharmaceuticals.
Arthritis Strength Tri-Buffered Bufferin is a trademark of Bristol-Myers Products.
Ascriptin is a trademark of Rorer Consumer Pharmaceuticals.
Ascriptin A/D is a trademark of Rorer Consumer Pharmaceuticals.
Bancap HC is a trademark of Forest Laboratories.
Capital is a trademark of Carnrick Laboratories, Inc.
Clinoril is a trademark of Merck, Sharpe, & Dohme, a division of Merck & Co., Inc.
Co-Gesic is a trademark of Central Pharmaceuticals.
Darvocet is a trademark of Eli Lilly Company.
Darvon is a trademark of Eli Lilly Company.
Darvon Compound is a trademark of Bristol-Myers Company.
Datril is a trademark of Bristol-Myers Products.
Daypro is a trademark of G. D. Searle & Co.
Disalcid is a trademark of 3M Riker.
Dolobid is a trademark of Merck, Sharpe, & Dohme, a division of Merck & Co., Inc.
Duocet is a trademark of Mason Pharmaceuticals, Inc.
Easprin is a trademark of Parke-Davis.
8-Hour Bayer Timed Release is a trademark of Glenbrook Laboratories.
Elavil is a trademark of Merck, Sharpe, & Dohme, a division of Merck & Co., Inc.
Emperin is a trademark of Burroughs-Wellcome Company.
Extra Strength Tri-Buffered Bufferin is a trademark of Bristol-Myers Products.
Felden is a trademark of Pfizer Laboratories, a division of Pfizer, Inc.
Flexeril is a trademark of Merck, Sharpe, & Dohme, a division of Merck & Co., Inc.
Indocin is a trademark of Merck, Sharpe, & Dohme, a division of Merck & Co., Inc.
Lodine is a trademark of Wyeth-Ayerst Laboratories.

Lorcet Plus is a trademark of Russ Pharmaceuticals, Inc.
Lortab is a trademark of Russ Pharmaceuticals, Inc.
Meclomen is a trademark of Parke-Davis.
Medipren is a trademark of McNeil Consumer Products.
Motrin is a trademark of The Upjohn Company.
Motrin IB is a trademark of The Upjohn Company.
Nalfon is a trademark of Dista Products Company, a division of Eli Lilly Company.
Naprosyn is a trademark of Syntex Laboratories, Inc.
Nuprin is a trademark of Bristol-Myers Products.
Orudis is a trademark of Wyeth-Ayerst Laboratories.
Panadol is a trademark of Glenbrook.
Parafon Forte is a trademark of McNeil Pharmaceuticals.
Percocet is a trademark of DuPont Pharmaceuticals.
Percodan is a trademark of DuPont Pharmaceuticals.
Phenaphen with Codeine is a trademark of A.H. Robbins Company, Inc.
Relafen is a trademark of SmithKline Beckman Corporation.
Robaxin is a trademark of A.H. Robbins Company, Inc.
Roxicodone is a trademark of Roxane Laboratories, Inc.
Rufen is a trademark of Boots Pharmaceuticals, Inc.
Salflex is a trademark of Carnrick Laboratories, Inc.
Skelaxin is a trademark of Carnrick Laboratories, Inc.
Soma is a trademark of Wallace Laboratories.
Talacen is a trademark of Winthrop Pharmaceuticals.
Talwin is a trademark of Winthrop Pharmaceuticals.
Telectin is a trademark of McNeil Pharmaceuticals.
Toradol is a trademark of Syntex Laboratories, Inc.
Trilisate is a trademark of The Purdue Frederick Company.
Tylenol is a trademark of McNeil Consumer Products.
Tylenol with Codeine is a trademark of McNeil Pharmaceuticals.
Tylox is a trademark of McNeil Pharmaceuticals.
Valium is a trademark of Roche Laboratories.
Vicodin is a trademark of Knoll Pharmaceuticals.
Voltaren is a trademark of Geigy Pharmaceuticals.
Wygesic is a trademark of Wyeth-Ayerst Laboratories.
Zorprin is a trademark of Boots-Flint, Inc.
Zyclone is a trademark of DuPont Pharmaceuticals.

# Contents

# Introduction

If you are reading this book, chances are that you or someone you care about lives with back pain. Did you know these facts?

- Most adults in America had back pain in the past year.
- Back pain is second only to the common cold as the most common cause of loss of work.
- Back pain is estimated to cost $50 billion to $70 billion each year.

*Winning with Back Pain* will show you that you DON'T have to live with back pain any more or suffer its effects. Using The 2-Week Plan to Relief outlined in this book, you can start today—right now—to control the pain and stiffness associated with back pain and look toward resuming your work and the recreational things you like to do—being with family and friends, sports activities, traveling—with renewed energy and enjoyment. All it takes is an understanding of the cause of your back pain; you can then begin to take charge with a treatment program that actually works. You can begin today to WIN with your back pain!

Back pain may last a few hours or many years. It may have a simple cause or a cause as serious as cancer. You can find the cause, learn specific ways to control the pain, and begin to prevent it from returning. The answers are here in this book.

You will learn the causes of *acute back pain* and how to make it go away quickly. You'll also learn how to deal with the back pain that lasts for months or years—*chronic back pain,* which can ruin jobs and make life miserable. As you start the basic treatment program outlined in this book, you'll be beginning to control the nightmare of chronic back pain.

This book gives you advice from experts on how to exercise properly to control back pain. You'll be given recommendations on medications that are best for easing back pain, and tips on how to prevent the pain from returning, whether at work, at play, or at home.

This book also gives you timely information on massage, acupuncture, spinal manipulation, surgery, and foods that can help treat back pain. You will receive advice on how to travel with back pain and ways to make the trip easier, pain-free, and more enjoyable.

*Winning with Back Pain* explains safety measures that prevent injuries at work and describes smart lifting that minimizes stress and strain on your back. We show you the devices that are available to give the back added support and strength when you must lift.

This book answers questions you may have about back pain. Here are some samples:

- Does treatment help back pain caused by thinning of the bones (osteoporosis)?
- Can future fractures from osteoporosis be prevented?
- How long does it take for the pain of a ruptured disc to improve?
- Does a ruptured disc have to be treated with surgery?
- How soon can I get relief from my back pain?
- Is prevention of back pain time-consuming or costly?
- What tests are available for finding the causes of back pain? Are these tests expensive or dangerous?

- Can stress affect my back pain?
- Are nonstandard treatments effective or harmful?

Start today to take control of your back pain by learning from the experts. If you have questions after reading this book, please write to the publisher, and your letter will be forwarded to one of the author-physicians for a reply.

Good luck as you take control and WIN with your back pain!

CHAPTER ONE

# You CAN Win with Back Pain

Back pain is such a common problem that most adults have experienced it at some time in their lives. Surveys indicate that in 1992 alone, over 50 percent of adults had back pain. With over 175 million adults in the United States, this percentage means that close to 90 million American people have back pain each year.

If you have ever felt back pain, you know how limiting it can be. It can be mild and last only a few minutes, or it can be severe and last for months or years.

Paul, a 29-year-old landscape architect, told us recently of how he was lifting some new shrubbery to show a client when he felt a fiery pain in his lower back.

"The shrubbery was light but now I feel hunched over and cannot walk without excruciating pain in my lower back."

Another patient, 63-year-old Sarah, came to our clinic with unbearable pain. "I picked up some boxes while moving last week," she said. "Ever since that day, I have been unable to stand, walk, or even sit without sharp pains in my back. What happened?"

John, a 44-year-old welder, told us of back pain that seemed inconsistent. "There is no rhyme or reason to my back pain," he complained. "I exercise and it goes away, then the next day when I sit and take it easy, it comes back. I do not understand this."

If you have suffered from back pain, you can probably empathize with these patients. In fact, the chances are four in five that you are like Paul, Sarah, and John, and have suffered this pain and stiffness at some time. Back pain sufferers are in great company: This common health problem affects people of every age, sex, and occupation, from those who do heavy labor to those who sit at desks.

Take Charles, for example. When Charles, age 32, was picking up his newborn out of her crib, he felt an excruciating pain in his lower back.

"I don't get it," he told us. "Here I run five miles a day, I work out with weights, and have no other health problems. Then I pick up an eight-pound infant and my back goes out. That makes no sense at all."

Back pain often works that way; unfortunately, it *doesn't* always make sense. It can happen at the most inconvenient times and often for the slightest reasons. Back pain can strike when you bend down to lift a heavy box or when you turn over in bed at night. Some patients tell of getting back pain when they bend over to kiss their children good-night or lean down to tie their shoes.

One older woman, who never had back pain before, bent down to pick up something from the floor and was unable to stand upright for the pain. Even though the statistics show that *80 percent of us have backaches* at some time in our lives, there is still good news. Low back pain is not normal, and almost all types can be treated successfully. You *can* win with back pain.

## The Cost of Back Pain

When 26-year-old Bill, a high school teacher, was released after a ten-day stay in the hospital for back surgery, he was shocked to receive a bill for over $18,000. "My insurance company will never cover all of this," he said. "What could I have done to prevent this expense?"

The cost of back pain is enormous, and prevention is important. This ailment has a high cost not only for individuals like Bill, but also for the nation. Many cases of back pain are not severe or long lasting, their treatment is not expensive, and job time is not lost. But when cases of back pain become severe enough to cause personal suffering and limit work, the cost of health care skyrockets. Studies estimate that the cost of back pain runs around *$50 billion–$75 billion* each year. And back pain is one of the most common causes of loss of work, second only to the common cold!

With these exorbitant costs and widespread suffering, it's important to focus on ways to control and prevent back pain. If only a small percentage of back pain could be prevented, the savings in pain and cost would still be tremendous.

## Is There an END to Back Pain?

What causes severe back pain? Can these attacks be prevented? What can be done when back pain continues for weeks, months, or years? Can the pain be stopped for good?

If you suffer from back pain, this book will show you how you can take control of the pain, stiffness, and limitation you are experiencing. You'll learn that you can begin to take steps *today* to prevent back pain from returning. If the simple guidelines given here are followed, your chances of improving and controlling back pain are good. You no longer have to just "hope it goes away." You can take charge of the pain and WIN with back pain.

## The First Step

The key to solving your back pain is to determine which kind of pain you have and identify its true causes. We see many patients who are frustrated because, after trying many treatments for back pain, they still suffer. Stores are full of remedies that promise relief for "back pain." Many other sources of treatment promise quick relief, but usually don't deliver it.

When many people talk about back pain, they really mean lower back pain in the lumbar spine, which is the most common complaint. The causes of back pain that we discuss can also affect the middle and upper parts of the back.

Unless you know the type of pain you have and the cause of your back pain has been properly diagnosed, you will have difficulty finding the right treatment. One single treatment cannot possibly relieve each of the hundreds of causes of back pain. The first step in finding relief for your acute or chronic back pain is to identify your particular type of pain and its specific cause, if possible. Chapter Two discusses this medical detective work in detail, but here is some general information and advice for all sufferers of back pain.

## Ask Your Doctor for Advice

If your pain is severe and is happening for the first time, ask your doctor for advice. If the pain does not lessen after a few days, or if the following important warning signs are present, make arrangements to get medical evaluation:

- The back pain is worse when you cough or sneeze.
- The back pain or numbness travels down one or both legs.
- The back pain awakens you from sleep.
- You have back pain and you find it difficult to pass urine or to have a bowel movement.
- Your back pain is accompanied by loss of control of urination or bowel movements.

These problems may be the earliest signs of nerve damage or other serious medical problems. You should seek immediate treatment for the best results. A range of different conditions may be creating these problems. Early and proper diagnosis is essential.

### Maintain a Positive Attitude

It may be hard to keep a positive attitude when you have back pain. The pain understandably wears down your resistance to feeling sorry for yourself and introduces many other difficult problems. One of your most powerful weapons against your problems is a strong, positive attitude. Your outlook on life and on your well-being is free and has no side effects. We can attest to the fact that the patients with back pain who have the best chance for recovery are those with an informed and positive attitude.

Become an expert about the causes and treatment of your own type of back pain. With that knowledge, you'll be able to manage your back pain in the same way you manage other areas of your life, and you'll get the best possible results.

In this book we will approach your back pain as we would in our clinic. We assume our patients are honestly interested in getting well. All the steps and guidelines are built on this basic assumption.

In some cases of back pain, the goal is not a cure, but it is reasonable to expect to be able to control the pain and stiffness. You should anticipate getting around and doing the things you would like to do in reasonable comfort. The good news is that most people can achieve improvement with back pain. It is very unusual to see patients who cannot be helped at all, even after years of severe pain.

## People ARE Winning with Their Back Pain

Winning with back pain is possible—many people are doing it. Remember, each case is different, and this book does not replace proper diagnosis and treatment. Talk with your doctor for specific advice in your own situation. Follow the steps outlined in this book, and join a happy crowd—those who have overcome their back pain.

CHAPTER TWO

# What Kind of Back Pain Do You Have?

Let's look at some of the most common types of back pain and the tests that can help with their diagnosis.

## Acute Back Pain

If you have ever had acute back pain, you know that it can seem unbearable. It can be a very sharp pain or a dull, aching pain. It is usually felt deep in the lower part of the back and can be more severe on the right side, or on the left, or in the center of the lower part of the back. Acute back pain sometimes comes and goes, but it is usually constant—only less severe or more severe. Acute back pain usually lasts from a few hours to a few weeks. One patient described acute back pain as feeling as though "someone put a blowtorch on my body."

Acute back pain sometimes comes on after an injury, but, more commonly, it has *no noticeable cause.* It may be made worse by coughing or sneezing, and its severity may wake you at night. The pain may be relieved by lying flat on your back—if you can find a comfortable position. Sitting in a chair can be very difficult and may intensify the pain.

The pain sometimes travels down one or both legs. (See Figure 2.1.) It can move down the front, sides, or back of either leg. When the pain travels down the back of one leg, it is often called sciatica. This name comes from the sciatic nerve, located at the back of the leg from the hip toward the foot. Numbness, tingling, or other sensations, traveling down the back of the leg along with the pain, can accompany this kind of back pain. One patient described sciatica as feeling "like hot water running down the back of the leg." The sensations of tingling and

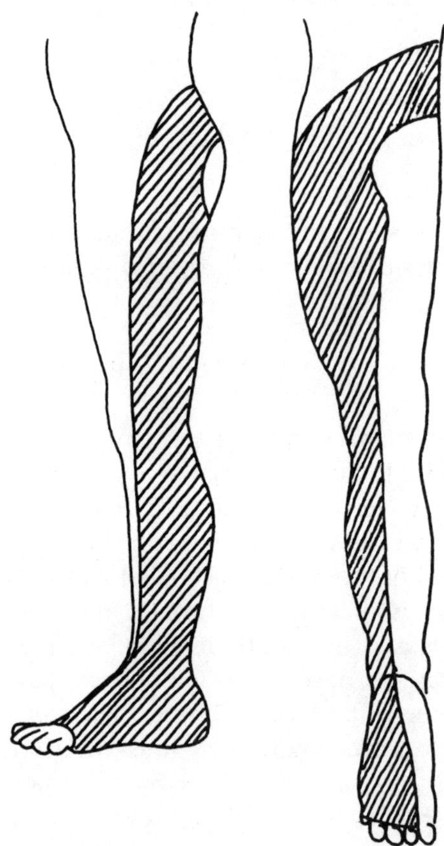

**Figure 2.1.** In sciatica, the pain may travel from the back down one or both legs.

numbness, and the pain, may become worse when you sneeze or cough.

Judy, one of our patients, told us that no one in her family believed that she was in pain because she looked so healthy.

"I fell down some stairs at a resort about a year ago and had some back trouble then, but after a little while, the pain went away," Judy said. "Then, last week, the same pain started over again—sharp and constant—on the lower right side of my back. My husband and children ignored my complaints and thought that I just wanted out of my housework. But I'm telling the truth; this pain is intense!"

Another patient, Felix, a courier, said he almost lost his job because of back pain. "My boss kept telling me it was all in my head. I almost felt as if I were a hypochondriac, until my physician ran some tests and verified what I knew to be true. My back hurt!"

Acute back pain is also commonly felt after an auto accident. The pain may or may not begin at the moment of the accident; it may begin and/or increase over days or even weeks, and finally become very severe.

When pain is the result of an auto accident, especially if the pain is delayed, questions arise over whether the pain is imagined or actually related to the accident. Because personal injury claims, lawsuits, and money are involved, proving the cause can be a very difficult problem to sort out. Chapter Ten discusses the problem of back pain after an injury or auto accident.

Unfortunately, acute back pain often begins with NO noticeable cause. The pain may be felt on awakening in the morning or may come on suddenly during the night. This pain may be puzzling when you are very sure that you have had no injury, fall, or unusual strain. This mysterious onslaught of back pain adds to patient's frustration. Most people assume that back pain must be "caused" by something that they have done. The truth is, sometimes the pain is there for no apparent reason.

For some people, acute back pain comes out of their past, not out of the blue. They remember experiencing the same kind of pain in a familiar pattern. We often hear that the pain is "like the old back pain." There may be familiar, repetitive situations that trigger the episodes of pain. Sometimes the pattern or environment of the attacks of pain can be a clue to their cause.

Because acute back pain is usually constant, you may have trouble standing, walking, or sitting. Simple daily tasks—showering, dressing, eating, sitting at a desk—may become impossible as the piercing pain limits your activity. Certain restful positions can cause you much more pain; others may give you some relief. It is important to try to find the cause of your pain, to determine the movements and positions that will make the pain worse or better over the long term.

## Finding the Causes of Acute Back Pain

The exact causes of acute back pain are often not traceable. Although a condition can be called acute lower back (lumbar) strain, the cause of the strain may be from an injury or may not be apparent at all. At times, there may be pressure on a nerve in the lower back. Specific medical problems can cause acute back pain, and it is important to find them. They include arthritis, fracture of one of the bones in the spine due to osteoporosis (thinning of the bones), infections around the spine, internal organ disease, and cancer.

Acute back pain can result from lifting too much weight at one time, but sometimes the pain happens just from leaning over, when there has been no lifting at all. One patient told us that his pain could come on if he leaned over to pick up a feather.

Another patient, Micah, age 26, had just given birth to her first child when the symptoms of acute back pain started. "I had no pain at all during my pregnancy," she told us during the visit. "I exercised each day, and even started exercising right after my baby was born. One day after I bent over to pick up a rattle, I felt sharp pains in my lower back. Picking up a baby's rattle caused this?"

Carl, a 46-year-old minister, was well and active until he got out of his van one day. "I don't know what I did, but when I pulled my leg around to climb out of the van, I felt an intense pain stab my lower back. Something serious must be wrong."

Acute back pain can happen at work. In fact, it is very common among workers who do repeated lifting, pulling, bending, or stooping. People who deal with heavy materials are at especially high risk.

Rob, age 48, didn't do heavy tasks at work, although his back pain was worse on the job. When he came into our clinic, he could hardly move. "I'm a drug representative for a pharmaceutical company. The heaviest thing I have to lift each day is my briefcase," he told us. "It isn't too heavy, but it is constant—picking it up, putting it back, then lifting it again before the next appointment. This pain came on suddenly last week and is so unbearable and constant that I don't know if I can go back to work."

Acute back pain can also result from a fall or other injury. Lower back pain is common after a person trips on a carpet or slips on a wet floor—so common, in fact, that "slip-and-fall injury" has become a popular description.

The pain may begin at the time of the injury or fall, but it may not start until a few hours or a few days later. The pain may gradually get more severe as hours or days pass. When the pain is delayed or gradually worsens over days, skeptics may wonder whether the patient is imagining the pain or creating some of its severity. Ask anyone with acute back pain: It is real, not imagined.

Most people with acute back pain, even severe cases, will improve or completely recover within six to eight weeks. During this recovery time, the steps we outline in Chapters Three, Four, and Five may help to shorten the span of pain and begin to prevent the pain from returning.

As we've discussed, the exact causes of acute back pain in most patients are not known. The disabling pain may start with or without a specific event that seemed to trigger it. In some cases, less severe attacks of pain over a few preceding months were ignored. Many patients are considered to have a "mechanical" back problem, referring to faulty coordination among the spine and the muscles, tendons, and ligaments around the spine. Even after extensive research, there are no definite clues to the exact cause of this common problem.

## Understanding the Trigger Points

Mac, a middle-aged college tennis coach, came to our clinic with acute back pain. He could not recall misusing his back in any way nor had he lifted a heavy object. Mac was very strong and healthy, but his back pain was keeping him from being active. He was found to have back pain caused by "trigger points" and started immediately to use the basic treatment plan outlined in this book. Within a period of two weeks, Mac was able to get back on the courts without much pain. Three months later, he was virtually pain-free, although he continued the treatment including exercise each day.

Like Mac, many patients have areas in their muscles and surrounding tissues that can produce severe pain. In this common pattern of acute back pain, localized points around certain muscles in the back and hips cause pain when pressure is applied. The pain caused by these "trigger points" can travel and produce pain in other areas. For example, a trigger point of pain around the hip may cause pain down the leg. (See Figure 2.2.) This problem of trigger points can accompany other causes of back pain or it may happen alone.

## Ruptured (Herniated) Disc

When acute back pain is severe and travels down one or both legs, the diagnosis may be lumbar disc disease. This is the most common cause of true sciatica.

Marian, a young preschool teacher, came to our clinic with acute back pain that was agonizing. "The pain seems to go all the way out my toes," she complained. "This all started after I leaned over to pick up a child out of her car seat. My concern is that it is intensifying each day, and I can't lift any of my preschoolers, much less do anything else strenuous."

After an exam to determine the problem, Marian was found to have a ruptured disc in her back. In rupture (herniation) of one of the discs between the bones of the lower (lumbar) spine, the disc material causes pressure on a nerve that extends down the leg. The disc rupture may also cause inflammation with swelling around the nerve. The pain is usually severe, as

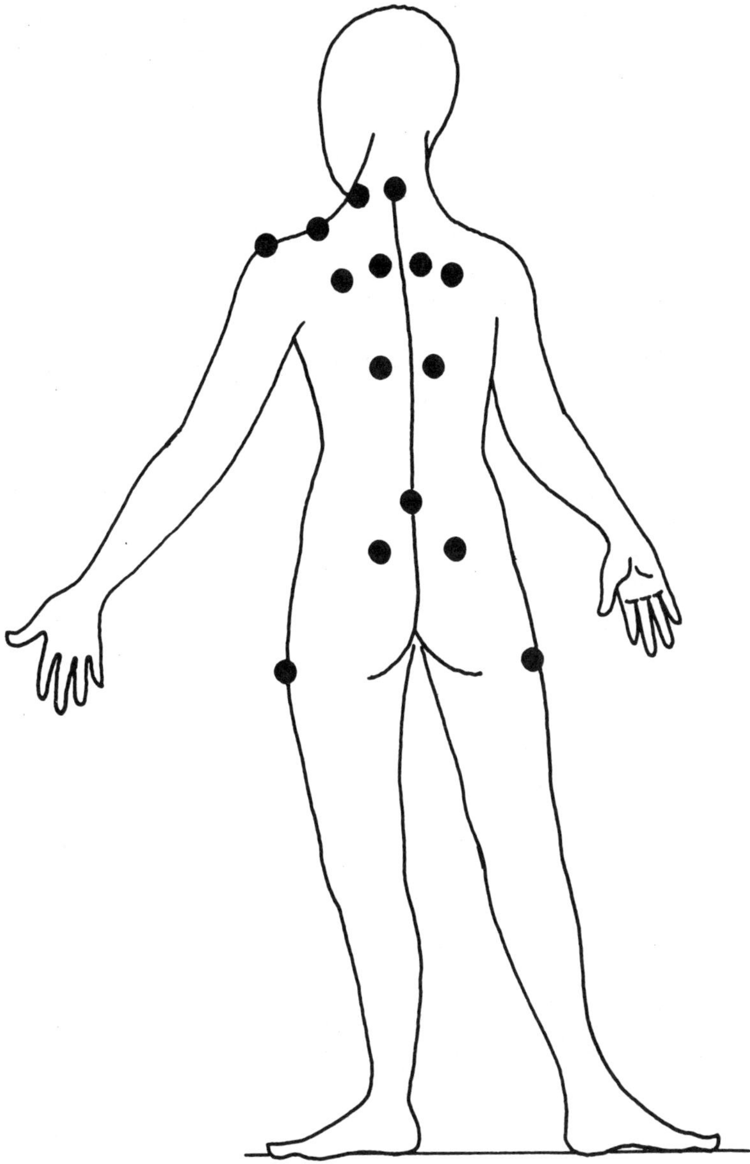

**Figure 2.2.** Trigger points are a common cause of back pain.

Marian said, and there may also be numbness or tingling. If the intense pain travels down the leg, it may cause weakness of certain muscles of the leg or foot.

As an example, a 40-year-old lineman for a utility company had acute lower back pain when he lifted a heavy load while twisting his body. The pain was severe and traveled down the left leg. He had numbness in the entire left leg and foot and was unable to sleep at night because of the lower back pain. The pain was worse when he sat in a chair and less intense when he stood up.

He found no improvement after treatment. Magnetic resonance imaging (MRI) showed a ruptured disc in the lower lumbar spine. (See Figure 2.3.) After failure to improve, he had surgery to remove the ruptured disc material. He has since had total relief of pain and has returned to work.

## Tests for Acute Back Pain

When is further testing needed? When the pain does not improve and activity or work becomes more limited, or when muscle weakness is found in a leg or foot, or when the bladder or bowel habits are affected. A diagnosis may be made after dis-

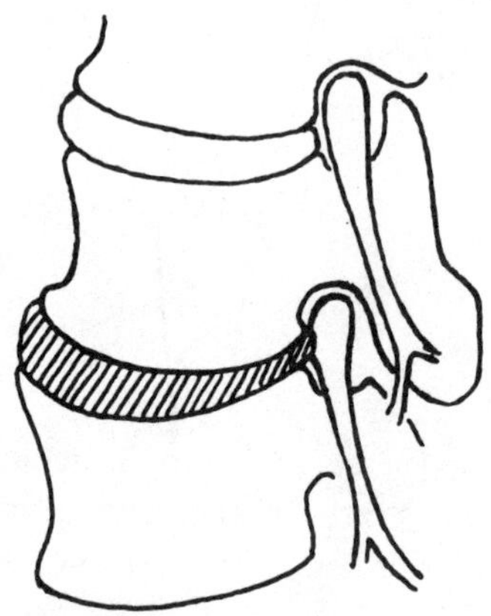

**Figure 2.3.** A herniated disc.

cussion and examination, and is usually confirmed by results of one or several tests.

If your acute back pain has not improved after the standard treatment explained in Chapter Three, further testing is also warranted.

These are the tests most commonly used for further evaluation:

- *X-Rays.* X-rays of the lower (lumbar) spine are an easy way to examine the bones in this area, but in most cases of acute back pain, these x-rays do not give the problem's answer. X-rays can detect cancer, fractures in the spine, arthritis, and some infections. X-rays are not able to detect a ruptured disc. (See Figure 2.4.)

  X-rays may not be necessary unless the pain persists. Refraining from using x-rays too quickly limits your exposure to radiation and your expense.
- *Computed Tomographic Scan.* A computed tomographic (CT) scan of the lower (lumbar) spine can detect the rupture or herniation of a disc in 75 percent or more of cases. Like most tests, CT is not perfect. This test may occasionally suggest an abnormality when the disc is actually normal. CT is better than x-ray for detecting other problems in the spine, such as infection, fracture, and cancer.

  A CT scan has an acceptable level of radiation exposure.
- *Magnetic Resonance Imaging.* Magnetic resonance imaging (MRI) is considered by most experts to be as good as or better than CT scan for detecting ruptured discs in the lower (lumbar) spine. It shows the ruptured disc accurately in 90 percent or more of cases and is not painful.

  MRI is more expensive then CT scan but does not have radiation exposure. Some problems may be found more easily using MRI, but, to diagnose some patients, CT or a combination of tests may be needed.

  MRI and CT scan can be done without admission to the hospital. Both tests can be done without injections

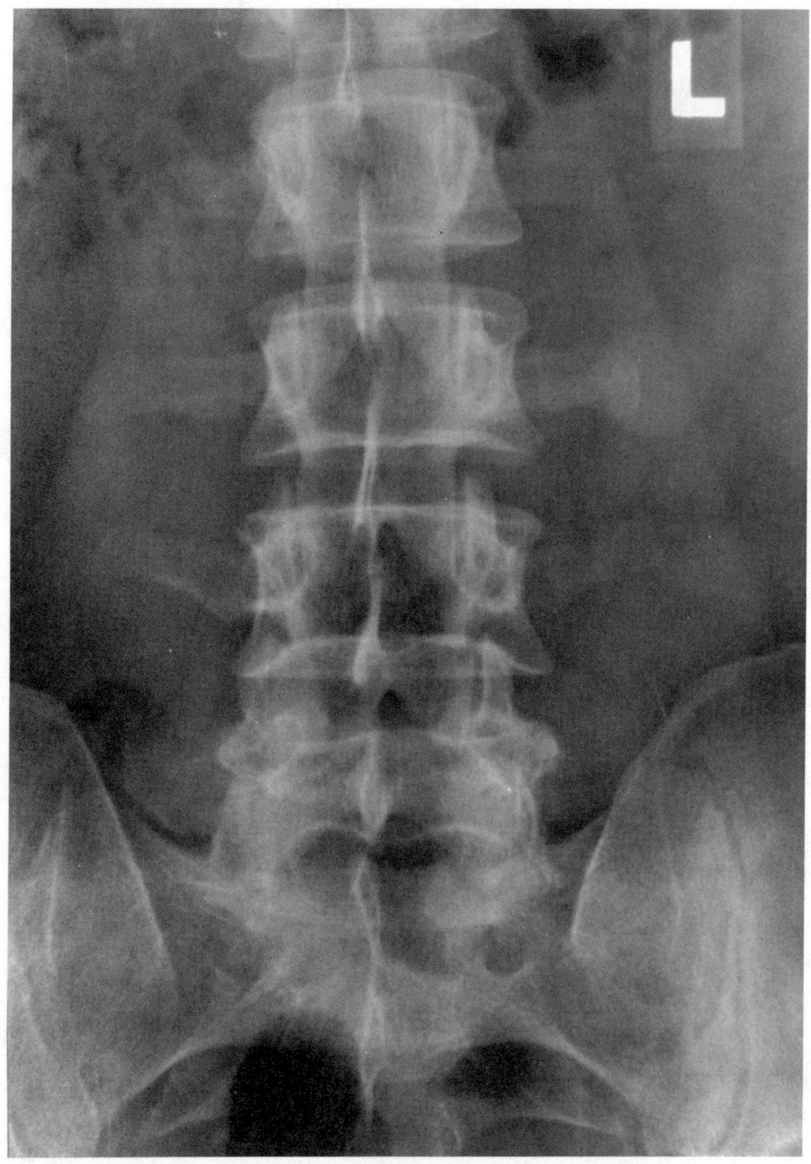


**Figure 2.4.** X-ray of the lower (lumbar) spine.

of medications or dye, and both have minimal risk. (See Figure 2.5.)

- *Myelogram.* Myelogram is a test that requires an injection of dye to show the rupture of a disc or other problems in the lumbar spine. It detects the rupture in over 90 percent of cases. Because it requires an injection, the myelogram has more discomfort and a higher possibility of unwanted side effects such as headache. Some experts now recommend MRI of the lumbar spine, with a myelogram performed only if the MRI does not give a clear answer.

  CT scan may be combined with myelogram to improve the accuracy of diagnosis.
- *Bone Scan.* A bone scan is a test that can detect abnormal areas in all bones of the body, including the spine. This test is used in some cases when there is suspicion of infection, cancer, or fracture. It does not replace the above tests but may add information by eliminating these other serious problems.

Other causes of pain in the back may be discovered by your doctor, often with the help of a consulting specialist such as an orthopedic surgeon or neurosurgeon. Each person is different and may require a different combination of tests. (See Figure 2.6.)

## Are There Other Causes of Acute Back Pain?

There are other, less common causes of acute back pain that you should know about. If you have any of the warning signs on page 4, you should talk with your doctor. If you also have weight loss, fever, severe pain in a bone, or pain in the abdomen, you should seek early medical evaluation.

Arthritis is one problem that can affect the back; fracture of the spine due to osteoporosis is another. Diseases of internal organs, such as cancer or infections around the spine, can also cause back pain. Some of these medical problems may not improve until they are treated—and early treatment is usually most effective in preventing future complications.

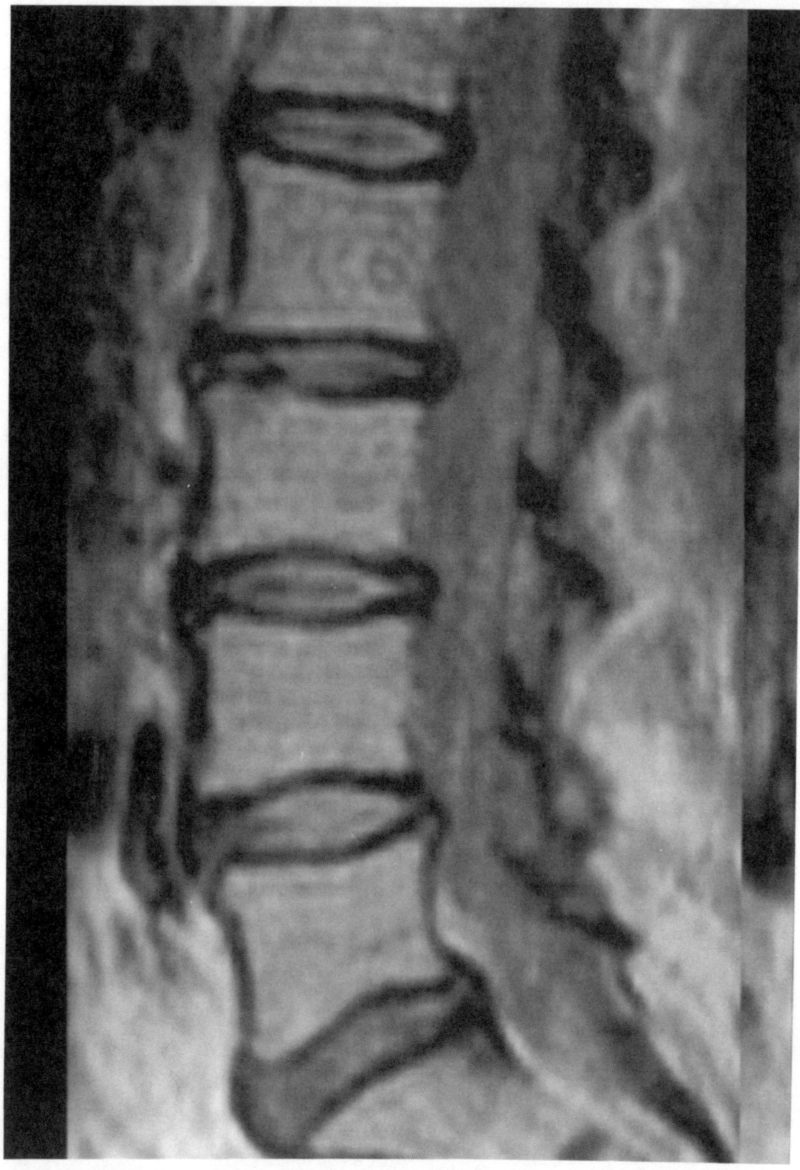

**Figure 2.5.** Magnetic resonance imaging (MRI) of lumbar spine.

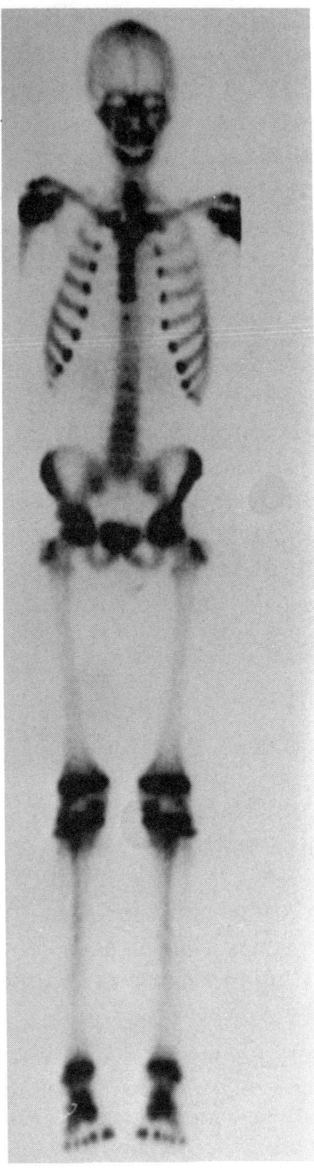

**Figure 2.6.** A bone scan is used when there is a suspicion of infection, fracture, or cancer.

For example, a fracture of a bone in the lower (lumbar) spine can cause severe acute back pain. This problem is most common in women over 50 years old, and the culprit is usually osteoporosis, which can now be treated. Early treatment can strengthen the bones and help *prevent* fractures in the hip, a common and dangerous injury among elderly people.*

We recently saw a 55-year-old woman who developed severe lower back pain after she had moved to Florida. She remembered no injury. She was found to have a fracture in one of the bones of the lower spine. (See Figure 2.7.) The fracture healed with only rest and her pain was controlled with medication. But osteoporosis was suspected as the cause of the fracture in the spine. Simple tests showed that the bones in her spine and hip were indeed thinner than normal. She began the effective treatment now available to try to strengthen bones all over the body. The treatment increases her chances of preventing a broken hip (hip fracture), which could be deadly, and of preventing another fracture in her spine, the source of her back pain.

## Chronic Back Pain

Chronic back pain is a pain that continues for a period of weeks or months with no relief. Fewer people suffer with chronic pain than with acute pain. Those who experience chronic back pain are in constant pain that is often severe. The pain might be less sharp than is acute back pain, but it becomes regular and nagging, and can be extremely limiting.

* A hip fracture usually requires a major operation, with major risk and expense, to repair the broken bone. The costs of hip fractures are over $7 billion each year. Up to 20 percent of older patients with hip fracture may die during the first year after the fracture, and up to 50 percent may require nursing-home care and may not walk as well after the fracture.

More prevention and treatment of osteoporosis could greatly decrease suffering and lower health care costs. See our other book, *Winning with Osteoporosis* (John Wiley & Sons, Inc.), for the latest information on osteoporosis prevention and treatment.

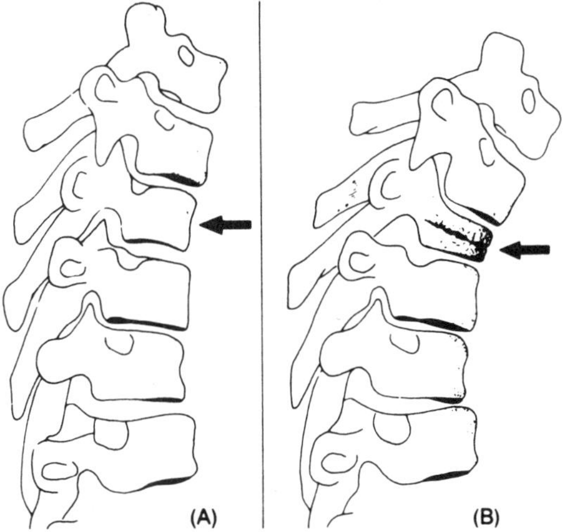


**Figure 2.7.** (A) Normal spine. (B) Spine with compression fracture. Note shortening of vertebra and abnormal curve of spine.

## How You Can Tell Whether You Have Chronic Back Pain

If you have chronic back pain, working may be difficult or impossible for you, even in jobs that do not require physical labor. Ordinary activities—driving a car, sitting, standing, and walking—may be accomplished in great discomfort, if they can be done at all. The pain is often much more bothersome at night and can cause you to lose sleep. One patient told us that she had not slept for days because the pain seemed to increase every night.

Chronic back pain can be a deep, aching, dull or burning pain. You might feel it in only one area, such as the lower (or middle or upper) back, or it may travel down one or both legs.

You may experience numbness, tingling, burning, or a "pins-and-needles" feeling in the legs. Ralph, a retired commercial fisherman, came to see us after having untreated back pain for over a year. Along with his severe pain, he felt a constant numbness in his right leg every day. Afraid that this numbness was a sign of a far more serious disease, Ralph became depressed and lethargic. He limited all activity in an effort to find a solution for his pain. Finally, when he could take the pain no more, he came to us for help in finding the cause of his pain. He is now well on the road to recovery and relief; he is now managing his pain.

When people with chronic back pain walk or stand for more than a few minutes, the pain usually worsens. Sitting may also increase the pain. Because many of their usual daily activities may be curtailed by pain, some people become virtual invalids. The pain can become a 24-hour presence with no break or interruption.

"I got to the point where I didn't want to wake up anymore, because I knew I had to face up to my pain," Miranda, a 29-year-old legal secretary said. "No matter what I did or how I slept, I had pain every morning, noon, and night."

Chronic back pain usually has an effect on overall attitude and disposition. Loss of sleep and loss of activity along with constant pain can make anyone more irritable and difficult to be around. Sarah, a middle-aged woman and mother of three children, told of how her chronic back pain almost ended her 20-year marriage.

"Before I started treatment, I was so irritable that no one could stand to be around me," she said during a visit. "My husband stayed at work late each evening, and the children would go to their rooms. I know I seemed cranky and mean, but I felt so awful—all the time. The pain began to control my life."

For people with chronic pain, tiredness and fatigue can become severe. Work becomes difficult, workdays are lost, and absences can extend into weeks or months. Some workers lose their jobs because of poor attendance, poor work quality, or a change in personality—all stemming from chronic back pain.

Even though fewer people suffer from chronic back pain than from acute back pain, 70 percent or more of the costs of all back pain come from the treatment and care of chronic back pain. If the total costs of back pain are $50 billion to $75 billion each year, think of the savings that would be possible from even a small improvement in chronic back pain.

If you have chronic back pain, you probably know firsthand how frustrating the search for relief can be. Walter, a 39-year-old retailer, told of meeting with six physicians before he found relief for his chronic pain. Many people will see ten or more physicians, chiropractors, and other practitioners in the hope that someone can miraculously end their affliction. Some try to achieve pain relief with standard pain medicines or will try stronger pain relievers or narcotics. These remedies give less than full relief and can be habit-forming, adding another problem—a dependence on pain relievers and drugs.

We have known many people who have had to start a treatment program not only to end their chronic back pain, but also to discontinue their drug addiction.

The longer the pattern of chronic pain goes on, the more difficult it is to change. With constant pain, many people become discouraged and depressed. The depression becomes a self-perpetuating problem and may require separate treatment. The feelings of the constant pain may become habits that are difficult to break. Some patients think about suicide rather than acknowledging that they must deal with severe pain and loss of activity for the future. We know of an older couple, both of whom suffered severe chronic back pain. Before they allowed proper treatment, they died in a murder-suicide.

## What Help Is Available?

If you have chronic pain, it is critical that you realize that there *is* help available. Remember, most people are able to gain control over their pain with proper diagnosis and treatment. You *can* manage and control chronic back pain. There is no magic wand to remove the pain completely, but, with treatment, the majority of patients find that THEY CAN GET AROUND AND DO THE THINGS THEY WANT TO IN REASONABLE COMFORT.

You can start today: End your chronic back pain by following the guidelines in Chapter Three.

## The Causes of Chronic Back Pain

Back pain is considered chronic when there is no relief after months of pain. Like acute back pain, chronic back pain requires an accurate diagnosis to determine the treatment that is most likely to help. There are so many "cures" available for back pain that some people spend years and thousands of dollars on remedies that promise results. The truth is, in most cases of chronic back pain, the treatment program described in this book will work in managing your pain. This treatment can be controlled by you at home and is not expensive.

If the pain becomes steady and limiting and is not relieved by the treatment measures outlined in Chapter Three, then you need more help. See your doctor.

If is not often necessary to have exhaustive tests performed. Usually, discussion, examination, and testing can lead to a working diagnosis that can allow a basic treatment program to begin. This will keep expenses to a minimum, limit your exposure to radiation, and spare you the many inconveniences of continued testing.

Once a specific cause of the chronic back pain is found, proper treatment can begin. For instance, kidney stones are one cause of chronic back pain. An elderly man came to see us recently, complaining of a nagging pain he had had in the right side of his back for several months. He had been taking an over-the-counter pain reliever, but the pain was still constant. After running a few tests, we found he had a kidney stone. Once this problem was taken care of, he had no more back pain. If you have a similar problem, removal or elimination of the stones by other treatment will end your back pain.

Other medical problems that can cause back pain require specific treatment that is different from standard back pain treatment. Some medical causes are not so obvious; for example, one less common cause of back pain is infection of a heart valve.

The main point is that correct diagnosis can resolve those cases of back pain that have specific or easily treatable causes. A correct diagnosis is the first step on the way to controlling chronic back pain.

## Can There Be More Than One Cause for Your Pain?

A correct diagnosis may find more than one cause of chronic back pain. This can be confusing, but patients who have had years of back pain may have a combination of some form of arthritis, pain in the muscles and other soft tissues, and a problem such as osteoporosis.

For these people, successful treatment must attack each separate cause of the back pain. When the basic treatment plan is started, it usually provides a measure of relief and allows the patient to resume daily activity with reasonable comfort.

We recently saw a 55-year-old woman who had had lower back pain for five years. She had gradually limited her activities and was able to walk only a few yards without terrible pain. She remembered no injury.

She was found to have arthritis in the lower (lumbar) spine, inflammation in the muscles and other tissues of the back, and a small fracture of the spine due to osteoporosis.

This is a common combination of problems, and, despite the complications, the treatment is not difficult and usually works well. The woman began a basic treatment program and, over a few months, had significant pain relief. She is now active, participates in a regular exercise program, and has resumed most of her daily activities.

A man in his mid-60s came to see us and said he could no longer ride in a car without severe lower back pain. He didn't notice this pain while standing, but when he was sitting down the pain became intense. The man loved to travel, and the pain was affecting his retirement activities. Upon examination and with certain tests, he was found to have arthritis in the lower spine. He began the treatment program outlined in this book, and, within just a few weeks, he was out in his car enjoying his travels.

Proper diagnosis allows effective treatment of the problems that cause chronic back pain. Even when your pain has been present over time, don't let discouragement and fatigue prevent you from receiving treatment that can give relief.

If the treatment you are receiving is directed at the wrong cause of your back pain, you will not have relief. What seems at first to be proper treatment can have delayed or poor results. Remember, if your treatment is not bringing improvement, it is possible that other factors may be causing your pain. Your doctor can help you uncover any untreated causes of the back pain and resolve them.

After discussion and examination, one or more of the tests described earlier will be needed. The computed tomographic (CT) scan, magnetic resonance imaging (MRI), myelogram, bone scan, or other tests may be needed to find the causes of your chronic back pain. Possible causes include a ruptured disc, as discussed above, or one of the problems listed in the following sections, or a combination of two or more causes.

## Arthritis

Arthritis is a common cause of chronic back pain. The type of arthritis most often related to back pain in general is osteoarthritis—often referred to as "wear-and-tear" arthritis, because it is more common as people get older or sustain injuries. Over years or after an injury, the cartilage between the joints of the lower back, spine, and hips wears away.

Osteoarthritis is a very common cause of chronic back pain. Osteoarthritis in the lower back can cause people pain and stiffness that worsen when they are standing and walking. You may have stiffness when you wake up in the morning and when you sit in one position for more than a few minutes. The pain does not usually travel down the legs. This form of arthritis may come on gradually and worsen over years. It may also worsen after injuries to the back.

Other types of arthritis can also cause chronic back pain. For example, one form of arthritis in the lower back, ankylosing spondylitis, especially affects young men.

A 25-year-old man recently came to see us because he had had pain and stiffness in the lower back for over eight years, and it was gradually worsening. On awakening in the morning, his back was stiff for about two hours; as he became more active, the stiffness decreased. He complained of milder aching in the shoulders and hips and noticed more pain when he sat at his office desk for prolonged periods of time.

The young man was found to have ankylosing spondylitis after x-rays showed typical changes in the lower back and sacroiliac joints. He began The 2-Week Plan for Relief as outlined in Chapter Three and over a few months noticed less pain and stiffness. He also found that his energy level increased. He now continues with a regular exercise program and a noncortisone anti-inflammatory drug (NSAID) for treatment of the arthritis.

Ankylosing spondylitis comes on gradually. By the time help is found, the condition has usually been present for months or years.

In this type of arthritis, the joints of the lower back—the sacroiliac joints and joints of the lumbar spine—become inflamed. Inflammation most commonly begins during the teen years and up to age 30. The pain may come and go at first and is often thought to be due to a strain or an injury. After a while, the pain stays and gradually worsens.

On arising in the morning, there is usually stiffness in the back that lasts a few minutes to several hours; there may be fatigue as well. Prolonged inactivity usually causes more pain and stiffness in the back. This type of arthritis is different from most back injuries, for which inactivity usually helps the pain.

With ankylosing spondylitis, there may be pain and stiffness in other areas, such as the shoulders, hips, or other joints. After a few years, there may be pain in the middle or upper part of the back. There may be a gradual stiffening of the spine and, eventually, of the neck.

Diagnosis of ankylosing spondylitis is usually made after discussion, examination, and evaluation of x-rays of the back. Other tests can be helpful. Proper treatment is especially important (and very effective) in prevention of deformity of the spine. For more information, see our other book, *Winning with Arthritis* (John Wiley & Sons, Inc.).

## Lumbar Stenosis

Another cause of chronic back pain is lumbar stenosis, a narrowing of the spinal canal that contains nerve roots coming from the spinal cord. It causes pressure on the nerves and, in many cases, pain is felt in both legs when the patient walks or engages in other mobile activity.

For people with lumbar stenosis, the pain often stops when their walking stops. Over time, the distance they can walk before they feel pain becomes shorter and shorter. This problem commonly happens in people with arthritis in the lower back, especially those with osteoarthritis.

We recently saw a 67-year-old woman who had felt pain in the lower back over the past year. She felt pain when she walked, and it traveled down the back of both legs. She found that when she walked a few blocks the pain started, but it stopped quickly when she rested. She was bothered by the fact that during the past year she had become able to walk only shorter and shorter distances. She had been very active and the problem was limiting her travel and volunteer work.

Magnetic resonance imaging (MRI) showed that she had lumbar stenosis. After surgery to remove the bone and other tissue causing pressure on the nerves, her pain was relieved and she is now walking without limitations.

## On-the-Job Injuries

Chronic back pain may follow job-related injuries. The most common causes of job-related back injuries are strain in the muscles, a ruptured disc in the lower (lumbar) spine, and a combination of "trigger areas" of pain around the muscles of the back and hips. (Tests for these conditions have been discussed earlier.)

Disability caused by these problems has greatly increased over the past 20 years. Although job-related injuries account for only 5 to 10 percent of the cases of back pain, the costs from this small group of patients account for up to 70 percent of the $50 billion to $75 billion spent on back pain each year.

Because of the high cost of chronic back pain with disability, it is important to decide the most likely causes in each patient and begin proper treatment as quickly as possible.

## Combined Causes of Pain

It is common to find osteoarthritis present along with another cause of back pain. The most common combination is with "trigger areas" of pain in and around the muscles of the back and hips. In many patients, the pain is severe, constant, and disabling. Diagnosis of this combination is made by finding arthritis changes on an x-ray of the spine and locating the typical trigger areas through an examination by your doctor. The treatment for each condition can be different, so this diagnosis is important. Both conditions need to be addressed in order for the pain to be properly controlled.

CHAPTER THREE

# The Basic Treatment for Self-Help

Once you have identified the type and cause of your back pain, you can focus on the fact that most back pain can be managed—if you use a basic treatment plan. In most cases of back pain, patients begin to notice relief *within 2 weeks* from the start of treatment.

Our 2-Week Plan for Relief, given on pages 54–57, lists the steps you can take each day to manage the pain and resume your usual activities. This basic plan is an effective beginning; by adding specific measures for your own situation, you can be sure that you are doing all you can to win with back pain. You can follow The 2-Week Plan for Relief for both acute and chronic back pain. If you carefully follow this 14-day aggressive strategy, you can WIN with pain as you take steps to heal your back.

## Treatment for Acute Back Pain

Believe it or not, most cases of acute back pain will improve with a few simple measures, and many cases improve without any specific treatments. When acute back pain strikes, if you have any of the warning signs on page 4, you should talk to a doctor to be sure there is no other serious problem present. If you do not have any of the warning symptoms, there are some steps you can take to shorten the pain and overcome the limitation.

Remember that the outlook for control of pain and for your return to work and activity is very favorable in the large majority of cases. Again, in MOST cases of back pain, patients feel relief within 2 weeks. You will too, if you diligently follow the treatment regime.

## Start with the Five Basic Steps

### 1. Limit Your Activity

If you have acute back pain, a reasonable first step is to *limit your activity* for a few days. Do only those things that you can do without severe pain. It has been found that, in most cases, many activities of daily living can be done without very much change in back pain.

If the pain with *every* activity is severe, try more limits at home (with more time in bed, if necessary, but not complete bed rest). Try to limit any bed rest to one or two days. Longer bed rest will not make most people improve any faster. If you have no pain relief at all, talk to your doctor.

### 2. Resume Activity Gradually

As soon as you can, begin to increase your activity. Standing, walking short distances, and completing some of your daily activities constitute a good start. Every few hours, be sure that you get up and move around for a few minutes. Gradually work up to activity sessions that are only 15 to 20 minutes apart. Then start to make each activity session longer until you have resumed most of your activities.

Avoid lifting, mopping, vacuuming, or other tasks that would cause more pain. A slight increase in discomfort is usually safe to put up with as you reintroduce your activities, but *if any action causes severe pain,* eliminate that specific action for a few days.

## 3. Apply Heat or Ice

For acute back pain, heat and ice may both be useful. With the use of heat, the pain and stiffness in the back muscles may improve temporarily. Heat can also be combined with exercises for comfort.

We suggest the use of *moist heat* twice daily, using one of the forms of moist heat listed in Figure 3.1. Use the moist heat for 15 to 20 minutes each morning and evening. Warm, moist towels may be necessary at first, until you are able to sit in a chair or on a stool (with rubber tips on the legs for safety) in the shower, tub, or whirlpool. Most people find the warm shower to be the quickest and easiest form of moist heat. To protect your skin from irritation or burns, make sure any moist heat you use is comfortable to touch. If the moist heat is uncomfortable even when its temperature is moderate, stop using it until you talk to your doctor.

Warm towels, or hot packs that can be found at your local pharmacy or medical supply store, are effective. Because some effort is needed in preparing the towels or packs, they may be slightly inconvenient. Some hot packs can be warmed in a microwave oven.

Moist heating pads are much easier to use, but they may not be as effective as other forms of moist heat when the pain is more severe. The pads may work well later on, after the pain has improved. (A dry heating pad is also easy to use, but moist heat is usually more effective.)

Heated pool
Warm shower
Warm bathtub
Warm, moist towels
Hydrocollator packs
Moist heating pads
Paraffin-mineral oil therapeutic mixture

**Figure 3.1.** Common Forms of Moist Heat.

The important thing is the effect—that is, improvement in pain. Use the form of heat that gives you the most relief and is also the easiest to prepare and apply.

Continue the moist heat twice daily until the pain improves, then decrease it to once daily if the pain allows. When the pain is gone, you may begin to use the heat only when you need pain relief.

Although most people we see respond better with heat, some feel more relief with the use of ice packs. With this method, ice packs should be applied to the area of back pain for 10 to 15 minutes several times each day. Ice may be especially helpful when pain is severe or is not relieved by heat.

Ice can be put in a plastic bag or standard ice bag, which is then applied to the painful area of the back. Be careful not to apply the ice directly to the skin.

Some people find more relief if they alternate ice with moist heat treatments. Choose the form of heat or the combination of heat and ice that works best for you.

## 4. Exercise

Yes, exercise can help end back pain. Most of our patients are surprised when exercises are suggested for back pain. We get this reaction because the traditional guidelines have often included prolonged rest and inactivity. But once the exercise program is begun, a majority of people experience improvement in pain and stiffness and a quicker return to activity and work.

*Exercise is one of the most important parts of the treatment of acute and chronic back pain.* Every day, we see patients who improve with a regular exercise program. Exercises should be done properly—carefully and slowly at first, then gradually growing in number and speed. This will increase the flexibility and strength of the back muscles. The support for the back is improved in turn.

One way to think about acute back pain is to compare the situation to that of an injured athlete. For an athlete to be prepared to return to the same activity as before, the area of an injured muscle or a strain must be stronger and more flexible than before. The only way to improve muscle strength is with exercise.

Studies support our statement that an exercise program usually improves acute back pain more quickly. In our clinic, the results of exercises begun early in cases of acute back pain are impressive. As part of the overall treatment program, proper exercise will allow an earlier return to work. Less cost and much less disability result.

It is important to start exercising very slowly with acute back pain. At first, when the pain is severe, the use of heat may make it easier to begin exercises. Using heat in combination with exercises helps reduce the pain and stiffness in the back. The use of moist heat for a few minutes just before or during exercise may make the exercises less painful and more effective.

The specific recommended exercises are shown in Chapter Four. It is best to strengthen all the muscles that support the back, including the back muscles and the muscles in the legs, ankles, and feet. The muscles of the upper body are also important for their support to the back. The stronger the muscles of the upper body, the easier walking, lifting, and other activities will become.

It may take you a few weeks to learn the exercises effectively and to be able to perform the correct number of repetitions twice daily. This perseverance requires your commitment to follow through with the program. The longer you do the exercises, the more benefit you will get; however, the benefits may not be obvious to you at first. Try to allow a *few weeks* of exercise before you expect to feel a difference in strength and flexibility.

You may need to begin with only one performance of the first exercise. Even then, there may be some discomfort in the back as you begin. (If you have severe pain while exercising, then stop immediately and call your physician for an evaluation.) After you have succeeded at one performance, at the next session try one or two repetitions. When you have mastered this number, try three or four repetitions and continue gradually increasing the number of exercises and repetitions. The goal is to eventually be able to do up to 20 of each exercise twice daily. For most patients, this is the level of exercise that seems to work well to maintain the highest level of strength and flexibility.

On some days, the exercises will be more painful than on others. Try to begin a regular program of exercise twice daily—on every day, good or bad. If you still have severe pain and can't do the exercises, then you should talk to your doctor.

### 5. Medications

Along with moist heat, exercises, and proper control of activity and rest, medications may help control acute back pain. In this situation, the medications do not cure the problem, but they give some relief while the other measures are taking effect. Try not to expect *total* pain relief, but do expect to be fairly comfortable. The pain reduction will allow more activity and will enable you to do more effective exercises. Medications should be taken only until the pain is controlled enough to get along without them.

In many cases, the pain can be controlled by medications available *over the counter.* These medications for pain include ibuprofen (Advil), aspirin, and acetaminophen. Follow the directions on the package label. (See Table 3.1 for common aspirin products.)

If you do not get enough pain relief from these medications, your doctor may prescribe one of a group of drugs

**Table 3.1**
**Some Common Aspirin Products**

| |
|---|
| Ascriptin (with Maalox) |
| Ascriptin A/D |
| Arthritis-Strength Ascriptin (with Maalox) |
| Arthritis-Strength Tri-Buffered Bufferin |
| Easprin (Enteric Coated Delayed-Release) |
| 8-Hour Bayer, Time-Release |
| Emperin |
| Extra Strength Tri-Buffered Bufferin |
| Zorpin (Zero-Order Release-Prolonged Action) |

called the *noncortisone (or nonsteroid) anti-inflammatory drugs.* These can help reduce the inflammation in the muscles and other soft tissues of the back. They also have a pain-relieving (analgesic) effect.

Over 20 of these anti-inflammatory medications are available (see Table 3.2). You should be able to find one that gives you satisfactory relief without side effects. Many of these products require a prescription from your doctor.

It is not possible to predict which of the medications will be the most effective. It is best to try a small supply for about

**Table 3.2**
**Some Common Noncortisone Anti-inflammatory Drugs***

| Trade Name | Generic Name |
|---|---|
| Advil | Ibuprofen |
| Anaprox | Naproxyn |
| Ansaid | Flurbiprofen |
| [Listing in Table 3.1] | Aspirin products |
| Clinoril | Sulindac |
| Daypro | |
| Disalcid | Salsalate |
| Dolobid | Diflunisal |
| Feldene | Piroxicam |
| Indocin | Indomethacin |
| Lodine | Etodolac |
| Meclomen | Meclofenamate |
| Nalfon | Fenoprofen |
| Naprosyn | Naproxyn |
| Orudis | Ketoprofen |
| Relafen | Nabumetone |
| Rufen | Ibuprofen |
| Salflex | Salsalate |
| Tolectin | Tolmetin |
| Trilisate | Choline Magnesium Sodium |
| Voltaren | Diclofenac |

* None is approved for use in pregnancy.

two weeks and judge the effect. This sampling can allow you to find the "correct" one for you. If there is no improvement or if side effects occur, then another should be tried. You can continue the one that gives the most pain relief.

Although most people do not have side effects, you should constantly watch for any upset stomach, nausea, heartburn, abdominal pain, change in the bowel habits, or other abdominal discomfort. If any of these occurs, report it to your physician. In this way, you can find the medication that gives the best relief with the least side effects. (See Table 3.3 for the most common possible side effects.)

If you take anti-inflammatory medications over a long period of time, be safe and check with your doctor at intervals for evaluation and blood tests.

Analgesics, a type of medication, may be needed simply to treat the pain associated with your back. There are times, especially before treatment is started, when ibuprofen (Advil) or acetaminophen in low doses can greatly improve comfort. Occasionally, stronger prescription pain medications are needed for short periods of time. These may include propoxyphene (Darvon) or codeine (often combined with acetaminophen or aspirin). (See Table 3.4 for the most common pain medications.) Propoxyphene, codeine, oxycodone, pentazocine, and hydrocodone should be used only when very necessary, to avoid becoming dependent on these drugs.

Other medications for pain that are available only by prescription include ketorolac (Toradol), which is actually an anti-inflammatory drug. Its advantage is that it may give pain relief without the use of a narcotic. It is used for up to five days at a time and can be given by injection as well as in tablet form. Your doctor can advise you according to your own situation.

*Muscle relaxants* may be used for muscle spasms in the lower back in acute back pain. Some of those most commonly used are listed in Table 3.5. A muscle relaxant may be helpful at night to improve sleep. These medications may cause drowsiness and require a prescription from your doctor. If no muscle spasm is present, these products may not give any further relief from back pain.

**Table 3.3**
**Some Side Effects of NSAIDs**

| |
|---|
| Indigestion |
| Heartburn |
| Abdominal pain |
| Gastritis |
| Peptic ulcer |
| Intestinal bleeding |
| Diarrhea |
| Constipation |
| Lowered hemoglobin (anemia) |
| Possible decrease in platelet effect (important in blood clotting) |
| Sodium retention with edema (swelling) |
| Increased blood pressure (hypertension) |
| Abnormal liver tests (blood tests) |
| Initial or aggravated kidney (renal) failure |
| Rash |
| Itching |
| Asthma (in allergic people) |
| Mouth ulcers |
| Palpitations |
| Dizziness |
| Ringing in the ears (tinnitus) |
| Sleepiness |
| Occasional blurred vision |
| Headaches |
| Confusion |
| Impaired thinking |
| Difficulty sleeping |
| Depression |
| Fatigue |
| Lowered white-cell count (blood tests) |
| Diminished effect of diuretics |
| Conflicting effect with other medications |
| Sun sensitivity |
| Meningitis-like illness (rare) |
| Other individual allergic or unusual reactions |

**Table 3.4**
**Common Pain Medications**

| Trade Name | Generic Name |
|---|---|
| Advil | Ibuprofen* |
| Aspirin | Aspirin products |
| Tylenol, Anacin-3, Datril, Panadol | Acetaminophen |
| Nalfon | Fenoprofen* |
| Ansaid | Flurbiprofen* |
| Combined with other medications | Codeine** |
| Darvon | Propoxyphene† |
| Roxicodone | Oxycodone‡ |
| Talwin | Pentazocine‡ |
| Anexsia | Hydrocodone‡ |

* Also can be used as an anti-inflammatory drug.
** Codeine is commonly combined with acetaminophen as Tylenol #3, Phenaphen #3, Capital and Codeine.
† Propoxyphene is commonly combined with acetaminophen as Darvocet or Wygesic, or with aspirin as Darvon Compound.
‡ Should not be used in combination with an anti-inflammatory drug without your physician's advice.
‡ Oxycodone is commonly combined with acetaminophen as Percodet, Roxicet, or Tylox, or combined with aspirin as Percodan.
‡ Pentazocine is commonly combined with acetaminophen as Talacen or with aspirin as Talwin Compound.
‡ Hydrocodone is commonly combined with acetaminophen as Anexsia, Bancap HC, Co-Gexic, Duocet, Lorcet Plus, Lortab, Vicodin, or Zydone.

**Table 3.5**
**Some Common Muscle Relaxants**

| Trade Name | Generic Name |
|---|---|
| Flexeril | Cyclobenzaprine |
| Parafon Forte | Chlorzoxazone |
| Robaxin | Methocarbamol |
| Skelaxin | Metaxalone |
| Soma | Carisoprodol |
| Valium | Diazepam |

## What about Rest?

Rest, including bed rest, is probably one of the oldest treatments for acute back pain. Even a few years ago, many persons with acute back pain were sent to bed for weeks at a time. This seemed reasonable at first, but when researchers looked more closely, they found that in most patients with acute back pain, bed rest helped very little. In many cases, it seemed to make things worse!

Staying in bed adds to muscle weakness. A normal person who goes to bed for one to two weeks is likely to become weak from loss of muscle tone and loss of conditioning. Instead of building stronger muscles to help protect the back, bed rest makes the muscles become weaker. A vicious cycle may be started, and the result may be more limitation, weakness, and pain.

Studies of people with acute back pain have found that the longer an employee remains out of work and at bedrest, the less the chance that he or she will return to work. If a person misses three months or more of work, the chances of *ever* returning to work go down alarmingly. In other words, the faster you are able to return to work, the better—and the less chance that you will suffer a long-term disability. Remember, most of the total health costs of back pain are incurred by the small percentage of people who become disabled.

### Combination Treatment May Be the Best

With a combination of proper limitation of activities, gradual increase in exercise, moist heat or ice, and medication, most people with acute back pain find the needed relief within two weeks, and almost all recover after six weeks.

### Will the Pain Return?

Whether the acute back pain will return in the future depends on the cause and other factors. Unfortunately, the cause of acute back pain in most cases is not known. "Mechanical" back problems or trigger points are often blamed, as discussed on pages 12 and 13. These attacks return in 50 to 75 percent of cases.

The reasons for the repeat attacks are not known. Sometimes, they seem to be brought on by lifting or other activity; more often, they have no apparent reason. There often seems to be *no cause* for the next attack.

The most typical pattern is for the attacks to occur one or a few times per year and last a few days to a few weeks. During the attack, the patient may be bedridden because of pain, unless the basic treatment plan is followed. The attacks may come closer together and may last longer at each occurrence.

Can anything be done to prevent the next attack? Some steps that may help are available. They are discussed in Chapter Five.

## Other Treatments Available

### Massage

Massage of the muscles, tendons, and other "soft tissues" of the back can be very helpful. Gentle rubbing and a "rubdown" at home can relieve painful and stiff muscles. If this cannot be done as needed at home, you may want to see a massage therapist.

Find a licensed professional massage therapist who has training and experience. Good massage can give relief that lasts hours to days. Massage can greatly help your treatment program by allowing your exercises to be easier and more effective.

### Manipulation

Spinal manipulation for back pain has been practiced for several thousand years. Hippocrates, the father of medicine, used spinal manipulation for treatment of his patients. Over the centuries, treatment in which manual manipulation is used has led to the development of chiropractic and osteopathy.

Spinal manipulation (sometimes referred to as spinal adjustments, by chiropractors) attempts to relieve pain by increasing the mobility between spinal vertebrae that have become abnormally restricted or "locked" and/or slightly malpositioned (subluxation).

After taking an appropriate medical history and performing a physical examination, the doctor of chiropractic, osteopathy, or medicine additionally palpates the spine to detect areas of restricted movement between vertebrae. Then, by applying specific manipulative procedures by hand, the doctor attempts to restore the lost mobility to the joint, thus allowing the vertebrae to settle into the most normal and natural position for them. The manipulations can range from a gentle stretching or pressure maneuver to multiple repeated motions at the same area or to specific high-velocity thrusts to affect the joints properly.

Patients may sense anything from a stretch or pressure sensation to a slight popping sensation as the vertebral motion and position are corrected. As with most physical medicine procedures, the doctor may prescribe that you have a series of manipulations performed until maximum relief is obtained.

These are some of the ways in which spinal manipulation works to decrease back pain:

1. Improves the mobility between two or more vertebrae, thereby reducing the temporary inflammation that occurs as a result of the locked spinal joint.
2. Often, reduces nerve irritation as a result of the improved mobility.
3. Allows surrounding soft tissues—including, but not limited to, the smaller spinal muscles attaching one vertebrae to another—to relax, thus reducing spasm and the pain that accompanies spasm.
4. According to some studies, manipulation causes the body to temporarily release endorphin, a pain-relieving chemical manufactured in the body.

There may be some temporary increase in back pain after the manipulation procedure, but that usually passes and the patient finds relief from the pain. Many patients note immediate relief after the treatment, without any exacerbation of their pain. If the pain continues to worsen after subsequent manipulations, the doctor will usually re-evaluate the condition before proceeding.

Manipulation is typically not done when the treating doctor determines that there is fracture, infection, cancer, severe arthritis, or other possible conditions that would contraindicate its use. As with other treatments discussed, there is no definite proof that regular spinal manipulation prevents future attacks or cures the acute back pain problem. But, for some patients, a periodic evaluation by doctors skilled in manipulation for the detection of any potential problems is part of their total health care plan, along with their regular physical examinations and dental checkups. Additionally, some patients once treated with manipulation never have problems again with the treated area of their spine.

Patients who get significant relief from spinal manipulation find that it helps them to continue with their basic treatment plan of heat and exercises, and allows them to resume a more normal life-style. Spinal manipulation by their doctor of chiropractic, osteopathy, or medicine may be part of a total team approach to the treatment of some of the more chronic, permanent spinal conditions. The skilled doctor of manipulation would then work in concert with a neurologist, orthopedic surgeon, or rheumatologist to bring about the best total results for that patient.

## Acupuncture

Acupuncture uses the insertion of fine-gauge needles into different selected points on the body to try to bring relief in cases of back pain and other ailments. The origins of acupuncture go back thousands of years. It developed mostly in Asia, but then spread to other regions. Acupuncture is practiced today in the United States by doctors who have a degree in medicine, osteopathy, or chiropractic and have subsequently been trained in the science of acupuncture.

Traditional Asian acupuncturists place the needles into specific acupuncture points along the body on lines known as meridians, to bring relief of patients' problems. Western doctors frequently utilize the same points, as well as local trigger points—knotted areas in a muscle that may be responsible for causing localized or referred pain.

Whichever method is used, you may find that a practitioner applying the acupuncture needles for treatment of back pain will select some local sites along the spine as well as some distant points on the arms or legs.

Western medicine's research into the subject tells us that acupuncture brings relief through certain reflexes in the body that occur by way of the nervous system. By stimulating one portion of the body and using pathways of the nervous system, an effect is obtained in the same or another portion of the body. Additionally, it is believed that acupuncture causes the body to release endorphins, the body's own pain-relieving chemicals.

You can expect an acupuncture treatment to consist of the placement of fine-gauge sterilized needles into the various points selected by the practitioner. The needles usually remain in place 15 to 30 minutes. The doctor may periodically stimulate the points by manually twisting the needles to obtain improved results. Another form of stimulating the acupuncture points once the needles are in place is to hook up the needles to small wires that are connected to a very slight electrical current. This procedure is known as electro-acupuncture.

There are ways of applying acupuncture that do not require needles. Using very sophisticated electronic equipment, the doctor can detect the local acupuncture point and treat it with electrical microcurrents. Some patients report good results with this method of acupuncture.

If you decide to try this science, you should expect a series of at least eight to ten acupuncture treatments, to try to ascertain whether the method will be effective for your particular condition. Acupuncture patients may gain no relief or may enjoy extremely long-lasting relief from pain. Always go to a *licensed* practitioner and make the practitioner aware of your entire health history.

Acupuncture has very few contraindications, and the side effects, if any, are minimal, but certain disorders such as easy bleeding and local infection may preclude a patient from receiving or continuing acupuncture treatments. You need not fear contamination from acupuncture needles. Practitioners use disposable needles and discard them after each application.

## Ultrasound

Your doctor or physical therapist has several methods available that can help ease acute back pain. In addition to hot packs, massage, and exercises, ultrasound treatments will help to decrease inflammation and may give additional pain relief. Ultrasound is safe when applied by a qualified therapist.

## Traction

Traction is an old method of treatment of back pain. The basic idea is to use weights to "pull" with traction on the lower back. This pulling stretches muscles and aims to relieve pain originating from the spine, discs, and soft tissues.

Some researchers have made improvements in the design of traction equipment, in an attempt to make it more effective. Many experts, however, have discontinued use of traction for back pain because it has not been shown to be very effective. Traction is best done in a hospital because the patient must stay in bed. This makes it a very expensive treatment for back pain, one that is usually reserved for only a few patients. Most patients find traction gives them more trouble than benefit.

## TENS

TENS (transcutaneous electrical nerve stimulation) is the use of electrical impulse to control pain. Electrodes are applied to the painful area and the electrical source can be controlled by the patient. This treatment is cumbersome because of the need to wear the device, and it can be expensive. (See Figure 3.2.)

Researchers have found that some patients gain relief with the use of TENS for back pain, but most studies have found less than major effectiveness. TENS can still be held available for patients who do not find relief with other treatments. Remember, TENS is simply pain control; it does not affect the underlying cause of the pain. If you try TENS, still keep up the basic treatment program to control back pain and

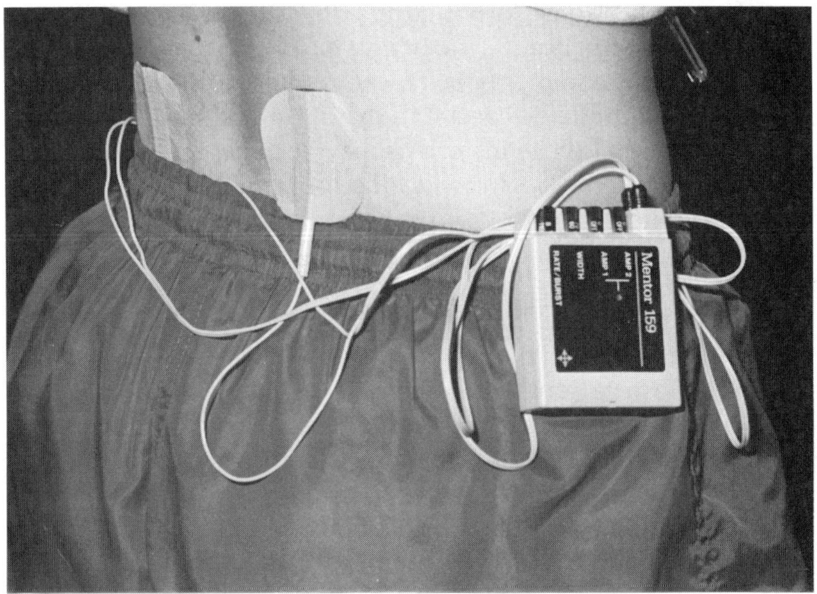


**Figure 3.2.** Some patients find relief with the use of TENS.

help to prevent its return. TENS is used more often in the treatment of chronic back pain than acute back pain.

## Injections

When trigger points are a cause of back pain, it may be possible to use a local injection for relief. The trigger point is injected with local anesthetic, which may give quick and effective relief. Unfortunately, the relief will not be permanent, but it may allow you to use other measures more easily.

For example, if the pain is relieved temporarily, you may be able to apply moist heat and do exercises more easily. These injections are safe and are easily done in your doctor's office.

Other injections are available for pain relief. Injections around the spine, called *epidural injections,* can be used, especially for constant severe pain that has not responded to other treatments. The injection is usually a combination of a local anesthetic and a cortisone derivative.

These injections do not cure a ruptured disc or a similar cause of back pain, but they may give pain relief. The effect is not permanent, but commonly lasts weeks or even a few months. If the duration of relief is excellent, the injection may be repeated, but be aware that these injections may be expensive, depending on your situation. You must decide for yourself whether your own pain relief is worth the trouble and expense.

## Back Braces

Back braces and corsets can be tried for acute back pain, but, to be effective, they may be heavy and can be very uncomfortable. Most patients find them so uncomfortable that they leave them off. If a brace or corset helps your acute pain, use it only as needed. Remove it when you exercise and as soon as you experience some improvement. Continued use of a back brace will not improve the strength of the back muscles, which is a major goal of the treatment and prevention of back pain.

## Surgery

If the basic treatment plan is not effective or gives only partial relief, surgery may be a useful consideration for acute back pain. The good news is that most people, even those with ruptured lumbar disc, improve without surgery. Researchers have shown that 80 to 90 percent of people with acute back pain can improve with medical treatment and can return to work *without* surgery.

A ruptured disc is the most common condition requiring surgery for back pain. As discussed on page 12, if the pain is intolerable and does not respond to treatment, or if muscle weakness or problems with the bladder or bowels occur, then surgery should be considered. Your doctor can arrange to get an opinion from an orthopedic surgeon or a neurosurgeon who can tell you your chances for success and relief of pain with surgery. Ask about the chances that your pain might *not* be relieved, and about the risks of the surgery.

Gather as many facts as possible, to be able to make the best decision for yourself. Ask for more than one consulting doctor's opinion, until you are confident that you have enough information. You should not feel rushed or allow yourself to be pressured about having back surgery.

The following different types of surgery are used to correct ruptured (herniated) lumbar disc:

- *Laminectomy and discectomy* remove a portion of the bone around the herniated disc and then remove the disc material.
- *Microsurgical discectomy,* which requires a smaller incision and microscope techniques, attempts to deal with a smaller area, risking less injury to surrounding tissues in the back.
- *Percutaneous discectomy* begins with a small incision that allows placement of an instrument into the disc space for removal of the disc.
- *Chemonucleolysis* is the injection of an enzyme (chymopapain) into a disc by a surgeon. The enzyme is supposed to dissolve the abnormal disc material. The potential side effects, such as reactions to the medication, and questions about its effectiveness in the treatment of a ruptured disc have made it less popular recently.

Each procedure may have an advantage for certain patients and may have less chance of response in others. Your surgeon is in the best position to choose the appropriate type of surgery. The factors that must be taken into account include your specific problem, the cost, and which procedure will best accomplish the goal.

When surgery is considered, you should discuss the planned type of surgery with your surgeon until you fully understand it and agree with the choice. You should feel comfortable that you have made the best arrangements for a favorable result.

## Chronic Back Pain

When your attacks of acute back pain come closer together until they are constant or become one attack that doesn't go away, you may have chronic back pain. Someone with chronic back pain is usually tired from the pain and lack of sleep it brings, frustrated at the poor result of treatment, and often difficult to be around.

The longer the back pain lasts, the more difficult it becomes to find relief and the less likely that a patient will be able to return to work. Remember that although chronic back pain patients are a small minority of all back pain patients, they create most of the annual expense of back pain. The sooner a patient with chronic back pain receives a comprehensive evaluation and begins treatment, the better the results are likely to be.

When your back pain is chronic, the first step is to be sure no other medical problems are present, as discussed on page 4. Tests may be needed to diagnose the specific causes of your back pain.

It is common to have more than one of the causes of back pain (see page 25). Among the most common complaints among patients with chronic back pain are pain in the muscles and other soft tissues, with or without trigger points, and arthritis, especially osteoarthritis. Pain that was present before an injury may be aggravated by the injury and become severe. In some patients, osteoporosis may be a factor and a fracture in the lumbar spine may be contributing to the pain.

Each of these problems has treatment available that may produce improvement in the chronic pain. Be sure that proper tests have been done to see whether surgery will be a benefit. For example, if lumbar stenosis is present, causing back pain when you walk, then surgery may be possible to relieve the pain. If total pain relief is not possible, at least one problem may be able to be attacked and resolved, removing a portion of the pain.

## Treatment for Chronic Back Pain

The initial treatment plan for chronic back pain is the same as for acute back pain: applications of moist heat twice daily, a regular exercise program, and medications to relieve pain. (See page 32.)

For chronic back pain, exercises are especially important. We find that those patients with chronic back pain who are able to do a regular exercise program are much more likely to improve, to resume their usual activity, and to return to work. Patients are often surprised at their own ability to exercise and increase their overall well-being. Try to allow a few weeks to two months to see results, after you start your exercise program.

We saw a federal marshal who considered retirement because of repeated attacks of severe back pain. The attacks could come on at any time, with or without activity. As is most common, no specific treatable cause of the attacks was found. He began a basic program including heat, exercise, and medications when needed, and continues to work with little limitation.

We commonly see patients who have had months or years of back pain but have never begun an exercise program. With help from a physical therapist and with proper care, these patients can gradually increase and maintain an exercise program at home.

## Add a Daily Walking Program

People with chronic back pain should add a *regular daily walking program* to the basic treatment program. Pick a distance that you can cover fairly easily, no matter how short. Then just gradually increase the distance as you can. (You may need to push yourself at first.) Most of our patients are surprised at how quickly their walking increases—and with it, their endurance, energy, and strength.

## Medications for Chronic Back Pain

Some of the medications used in acute back pain (see page 36) may also be helpful in chronic back pain. Among those that are most helpful are the group of *noncortisone or nonsteroid anti-inflammatory drugs.* These may be effective in helping to control any pain or inflammation that is present.

Another group of medications, used for years for other problems, can help the pain and stiffness of chronic back pain.

For example, antidepressants may have an anti-inflammatory effect and may help control the pain of chronic back pain. The response is sometimes excellent with relief from pain and stiffness, increased activity, and an improved nighttime sleep pattern. The response is usually seen over a period of several weeks. These medications may be most helpful when combined with one of the noncortisone anti-inflammatory drugs. (See page 37.) However, do *not* combine mediations unless recommended by your doctor.

The side effects of these "antidepressants" are usually minimal when dosage is low, but they can include mouth dryness, constipation, dizziness, palpitations (rapid or forceful heartbeat), or a calming (sedating) effect. At higher doses or in older people, difficulty in urination or blurred vision can result. If you have glaucoma or prostate problems, you should take these medications with special caution and only after you discuss your condition with your doctor. In some people, these medications produce weakness or fatigue. Fluid retention or cardiac problems can be aggravated, or tremors may occur, but usually at higher doses. In addition, allergic reactions can occur, as with any drug.

The use of narcotics for chronic back pain should be avoided as much as possible because of the possibility of dependence. They give little long-term relief but may be prescribed on occasion. Some of the nonnarcotic pain medications listed on page 40 may be helpful. Your doctor can help you, after evaluating your own situation.

## Managing Stress with Chronic Back Pain

The stress of living with constant pain is high. Researchers have found that, in chronic back pain, the role of stress and other psychological factors may be more important than the original cause or injury that created the pain. These nonphysical aspects of chronic back pain must be recognized and treated with the same attention given to any other part of the problem. In Chapter Eight, we'll discuss how you can manage the stress of chronic back pain.

## Pain Control Centers

If, after a reasonable time, you do not have adequate pain relief and improved activity, you should consider referral to a *major comprehensive pain center.* There, a team approach will attempt to deal with every aspect of your problem of chronic back pain.

There are a number of types of pain control clinics. Some use one type of pain relief, such as injections. Others concentrate on the stress and psychological aspects of pain control. Important parts of the management of chronic back pain are often (1) evaluation of depression from the pain, (2) teaching ways to cope with back pain, and (3) measurement of disability.

If you don't get enough relief after treatment, you should ask your doctor for a referral to a qualified comprehensive pain control center. All available techniques to thoroughly evaluate chronic back pain are used at this type of pain control center. Good centers are able to help the majority of people who go to them, even people who have had little pain relief for years.

# Your 2-Week Plan for Relief

Winning with back pain takes a great deal of initiative on your part as you undertake a vigorous treatment program. But the results of less pain and greater mobility will be well worth the time and effort this program demands. Most cases of back pain will respond to treatment within two weeks, if you diligently stick with the strategy explained here.

The 2-Week Plan for Relief is no substitute for medical care by your personal physician, but it is an effective treatment for most cases of back pain. Caution: Some cases of back pain require a physician's evaluation and special treatment. DO NOT use The 2-Week Plan for Relief if you have any of the warning signs listed on page 4. If in doubt, see your physician for a diagnosis, then begin The 2-Week Plan for Relief to end your back pain.

**WEEK I**
**Days 1–3**
**Morning**

- Rest as needed; allow only mild activity.
- Apply moist heat two or three times on painful area. (Sit in a warm tub of water, or sit on a stool or stand in the shower. Allow the warm water to hit the painful area for 10 to 15 minutes. A whirlpool is excellent if available. Warm towels can also work. (See page 33.)
- Take the medications as approved by your physician throughout the day and evening.
- Alternate moist heat with ice packs for 10 minutes, if ice helps the pain.
- Begin the exercise program when your back is feeling less painful. (Start slowly; do only one or two repetitions of a few of the exercises shown in Chapter Four. Stop if you feel any intense or unusual pain, and do not resume the exercise. Call your physician or physical therapist if necessary.)
- Start with a five-minute walk, if your pain is not severe.

**Noon**

- Rest as needed; allow mild activity.
- Use moist heat for one or two sessions, as in the morning.
- Try to walk for five minutes.
- Take medications as approved.

**Evening**

- Rest; allow mild activity.
- Apply moist heat for one or two sessions.

- Try to walk for five minutes, if you can do so without pain.
- Repeat the morning exercises, starting slowly (one or two repetitions of a few exercises). Stop if you feel any intense or unusual pain.

**Days 4–7**
**Morning**

- Start the morning with moist heat (shower, bathtub, whirlpool, or warm towels). Repeat once or twice, for 10 to 15 minutes in each session.
- Increase activity throughout the day, allowing for times of rest. Gradually, do more of your usual daily activities, but avoid lifting, bending, mopping, or vacuuming.
- Continue the exercise program you started on Day 1. (Remember to start slowly, doing only a few repetitions of each exercise. Gradually increase the exercises, but stop if you feel any intense or unusual pain. Call your physician or physical therapist if necessary.)

**Noon**

- Apply moist heat, then gradually increase your combination of activity and periods of rest. (A moist heating pad can be used as you sit at your desk. If possible on your lunch break, expose the injured area to a moist towel, a warm shower, or hot tub.)
- Walk for five minutes.

**Evening**

- Do some stretching exercises or isometrics after a 10- to 15-minute period of moist heat in the warm shower, bathtub, or whirlpool.

- Stay on any medications your physician has prescribed.

## WEEK II
### Days 8–11 (Greater Activity Days)
### Morning

- Start the day with a warm shower or bath. (Be sure painful areas are surrounded with this moist heat.)
- Do your exercises for stretching and strengthening, gradually increasing their number of repetitions.
- Take a five-minute walk. (Again, if your back has unusual or intense pain, call your physician for an evaluation.)

### Noon

- Continue the moist heat. Take a five-minute walk.
- Increase the exercise program to include all exercises in Chapter Four. Start with just a few repetitions on Day 8 and increase the repetitions as you are able to (without discomfort).

### Evening

- Soak in a warm tub, shower, or whirlpool bath.
- Take another five-minute walk.
- Do the back exercises, gradually increasing toward your goal of 20 repetitions of each exercise twice daily.

### Days 12–14 (Resuming Regular Activities Days)
### Morning

- Start your day with moist heat treatments.
- Take medications as directed by your physician.

- Continue the exercise program as outlined in Chapter Four.
- Try to increase your walking, if you can do so without pain. (If you are feeling more pain, go back to the treatment suggested for Days 4–7, then increase as you can.)

**Noon**

- Use a moist heating pad until you have no pain.
- Instead of sitting during lunch break, try to do some stretching exercises or isometrics as suggested in Chapter Four. (You may be stiff at first, but these exercises will help your flexibility.)
- Continue the five- or ten-minute walk daily at this time.

**Evening**

- Soak in a whirlpool bath or warm shower.
- Continue the exercises, working further toward your goal of 20 repetitions of each exercise twice daily.
- Increase your walk to 20 minutes, if you can do so without pain.
- If you are still feeling pain, you should see your doctor.

**Recovery**

If you follow this plan for a 2-week period, your back should be on its way to recovery. Don't forget to continue the exercise program every day as indicated in Chapter 4, and be sure to keep walking at the suggested times. IF you are still feeling pain, you may need an evaluation by your physician.

CHAPTER FOUR

# A Daily Exercise Program for Your Back

Exercise is the key for management of your back pain and for prevention of future pain. Exercises for the back strengthen the muscles, give the spine more support, and make the back more flexible and limber. For the most common causes of acute back pain, exercises can shorten the time of severe pain and disability. For many of the other causes of back pain, such as osteoporosis and many types of arthritis, exercise is a critical part of the basic treatment program.

In our clinic, we have found that:

- People with many types of back pain who can maintain a regular exercise program are able to see and feel improvement.
- People who do not use exercise as part of their treatment usually experience much less relief from the back pain.

When starting an exercise program, try to allow yourself time to get adjusted to the movements, to learn the exercises, and to condition your body to perform each exercise in a manner that will increase your strength. It usually takes several days or a few weeks to learn to do the exercises effectively and to be able to perform the maximum repetitions required twice daily. You need to make a commitment to start and *stay with* the program to achieve relief. Keep in mind that the exercises will take effect over a period of a few weeks to a few months—it takes time to build muscles.

Don't worry about your muscles being old or out of condition. Begin slowly, with only one or two repetitions of each exercise twice daily—usually in the morning and evening. Gradually increase until you can work up to 10, 15, and finally 20 repetitions of each exercise twice daily.

If you have more pain after you exercise than before, you may need to go more slowly, doing only one or two repetitions of the first exercise once a day and gradually increasing. You may find it easier to do the exercises just after you apply moist heat, when the muscles are looser and more flexible. It may help to do the exercises in the shower or in a warm bath or whirlpool.

You should have no more pain after you finish than when you started your exercises. If you have severe pain while exercising, you should stop. At the next session, try one or two repetitions of the exercises again. When you have mastered this number, try three or four repetitions, gradually increasing the number of repetitions and exercises. The goal—up to 20 of each exercise twice daily—is the level that seems to work best to maintain a good level of strength and flexibility.

On days when you are uncomfortable or tired, you will not feel like exercising. But you must maintain the twice-daily schedule on good days and on bad days, to achieve maximum improvement. When you improve, in a few weeks to a few months, *don't stop the exercises.*

It may be helpful to begin your exercise program with the help and instruction of a physical therapist. The therapist can be sure you are doing the exercises correctly so that you get the maximum benefit. The therapist can also instruct you in the proper positioning of moist heat, hot packs, and other helpful treatment. When you can perform the exercises as effectively at home as with the therapist, you can maintain the program at home, seeing the therapist only as needed. Ask your doctor for a referral to a certified therapist in your community.

Let's review the specific exercises that can allow you to maintain joint flexibility and muscle strength.

## Exercises for Neck Mobility and Flexibility

These exercises improve the mobility and flexibility of the neck. Flexibility helps your body perform more effectively. You may do these exercises sitting or standing, whichever is more comfortable for you. Some people like to do these exercises in front of a mirror.

Keep your head straight and looking forward. Try to achieve the most movement possible with the range-of-motion exercises. Then try the isometric strengthening exercises. You should begin these with minimal resistance, very gradually increasing the resistance as you are able. Sometimes it is helpful to have some gentle assistance from a family member or friend. Your physical therapist can show you how.

### Range-of-Motion Neck Exercises

*Flexion.* Look down and bend your chin forward to the chest (see Figure 4.1). If you feel stiffness or pain, do not force the movement. Go as far as you can move easily. If your back pain worsens with this or any exercise, then stop until you have talked to your physician or physical therapist.

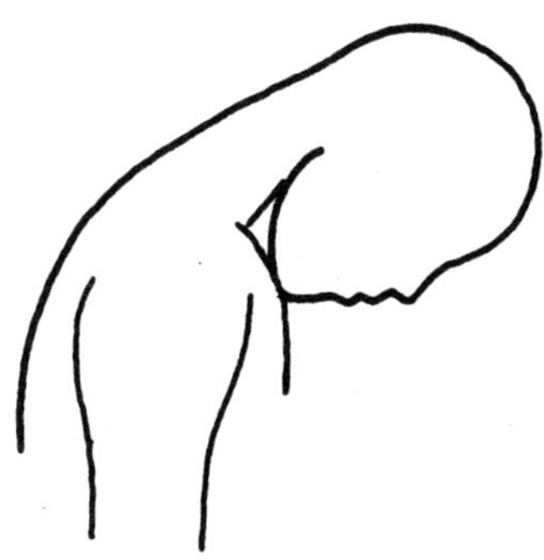

**Figure 4.1.** A flexion exercise.

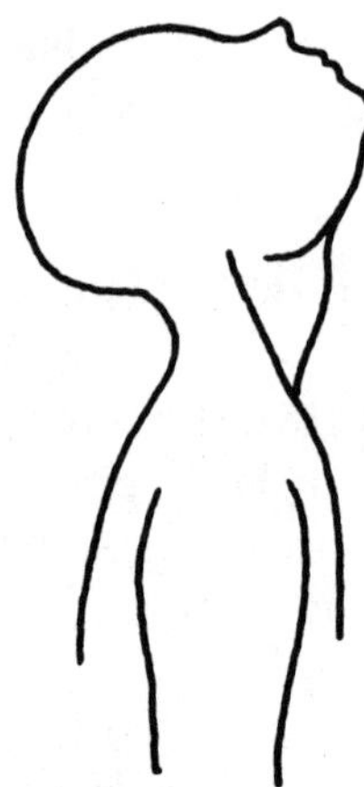

**Figure 4.2.** An extension exercise.

*Extension.* Look up and bend your head back as far as possible without forcing any movement (see Figure 4.2). If you feel pain or dizziness, stop until you talk to your physician or physical therapist.

*Lateral Flexion.* Tilt your left ear to your left shoulder (but do not raise the shoulder). If you feel pain or resistance, do not force the motion.

Now tilt the right ear to the right shoulder just as you did for the left ear (see Figure 4.3).

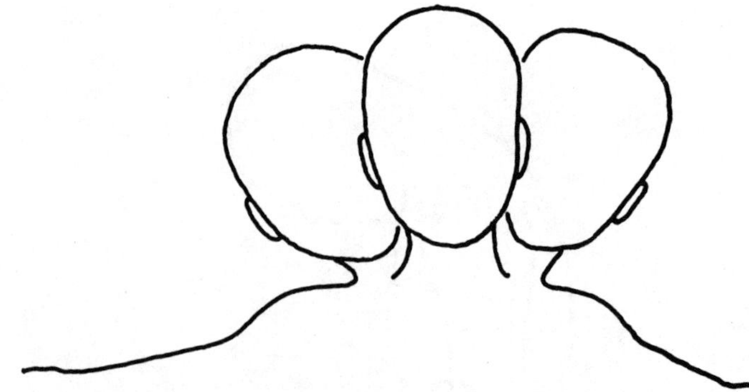

**Figure 4.3.** A lateral flexion exercise.

*Rotation.* Turn to look over your left shoulder. Try to make your chin even with your shoulder. Go as far as is comfortable, but do not force the movement (see Figure 4.4).

Now turn and look over your right shoulder, just as you did over your left shoulder.

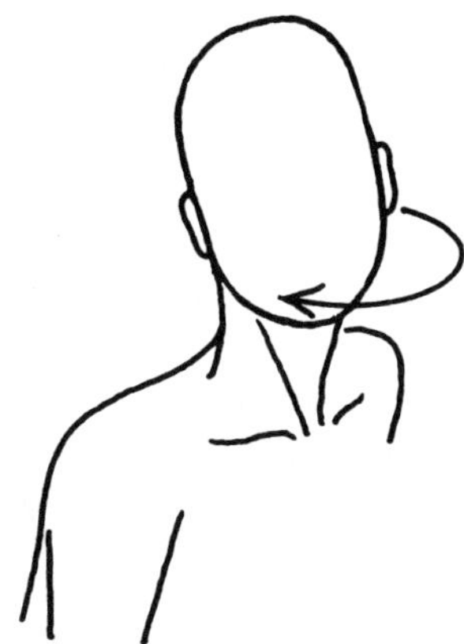

**Figure 4.4.** A rotation exercise.

## Neck Isometric Exercises

Neck isometric exercises are more advanced exercises to help strengthen the muscles of the neck. Try these gently and gradually after the range of motion of your neck is improved as much as possible.

*Isometric Flexion.* Place your hand on your forehead. Try to look down while resisting the motion with your hand. Hold for six seconds. Count out loud. Do NOT hold your breath. (See Figure 4.5.)

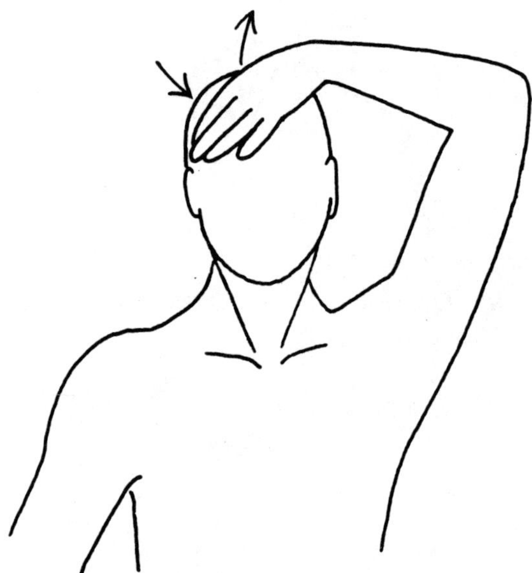

**Figure 4.5.** An isometric flexion exercise.

*Isometric Extension.* Place your hands on the back of your head (see Figure 4.6). Try to look up and back while resisting the motion with your hands. Hold for six seconds. Count out loud. Do NOT hold your breath.

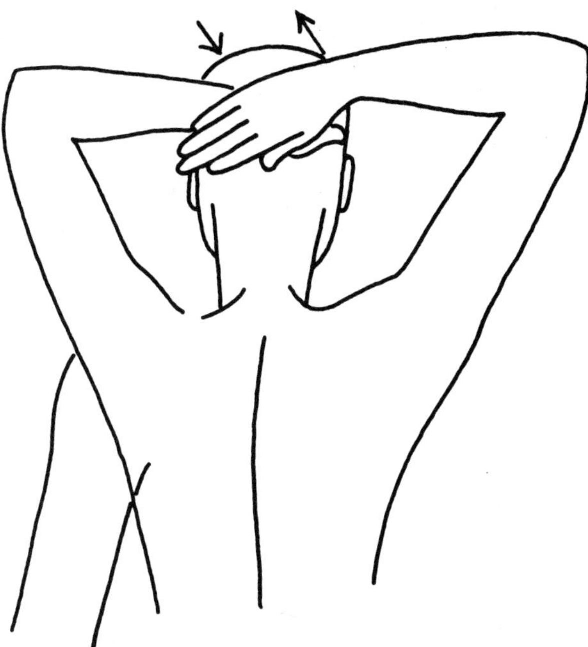

**Figure 4.6.** An isometric extension exercise.

*Isometric Lateral Flexion.* Start with your head straight. Place your left hand just above your left ear (see Figure 4.7). Try to tilt your head to the left but resist the motion with your left hand. Hold for six seconds. Count out loud. Do NOT hold your breath.

Now place your right hand just above your right ear. Try to tilt your head to the right but resist the movement with your right hand. Hold for six seconds. Count out loud. Do NOT hold your breath.

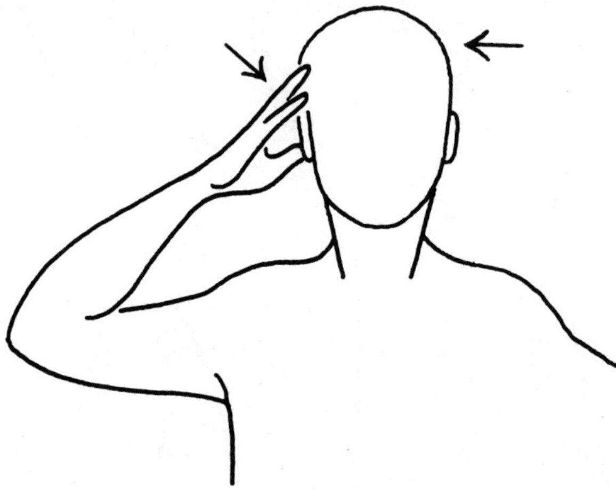

**Figure 4.7.** An isometric lateral flexion exercise.

*Isometric Rotation.* Place your left hand above your ear and near your left forehead (see Figure 4.8). Now try to look over your left shoulder but resist the motion with your left hand. (The hand should not be placed on the jaw.) Hold for six seconds. Count out loud. Do NOT hold your breath.

Now place your right hand above your ear and near your right forehead. Try to look over your right shoulder but resist the motion with your right hand. Hold for six seconds. Count out loud. Do NOT hold your breath.

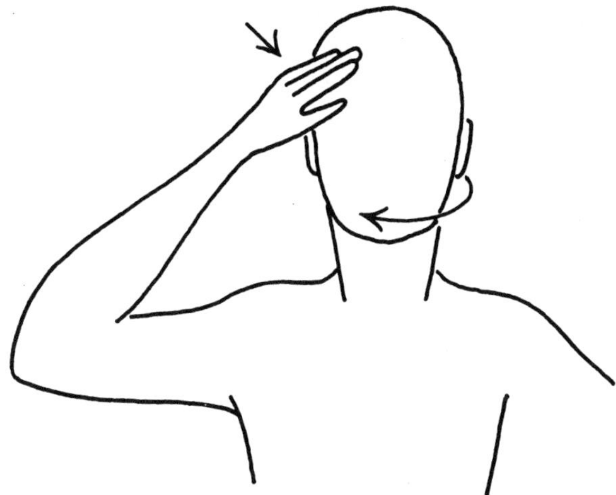

**Figure 4.8.** An isometric rotation exercise.

## Shoulder Flexibility Exercises

These exercises will increase the flexibility of the shoulders and arms. Increasing the number of exercises can increase the strength of the arms.

### Shoulder External Rotation

These exercises increase the motion you use to comb your hair. You may sit, stand, or lie down to do these exercises. (See Figure 4.9.)

Clasp your hands behind your head. Pull your elbows together until they are as close as possible in front of your chin. Separate the elbows to the side as much as possible.

Repeat this, gradually increasing to five, then more, up to 20 repetitions. You may repeat these movements two or three times daily.

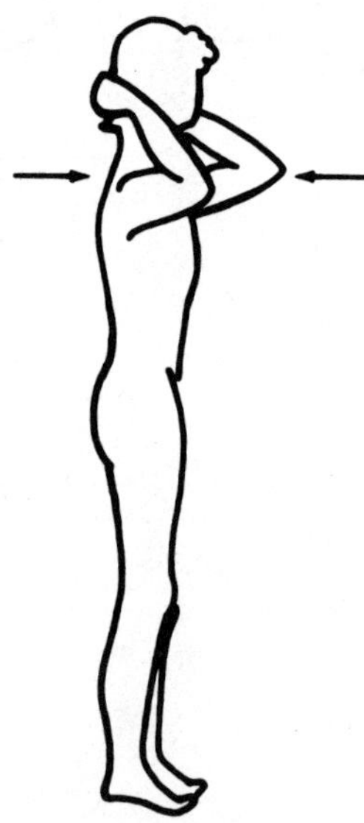

**Figure 4.9.** An external rotation exercise.

## Shoulder Internal Rotation

These exercises increase the flexibility of the shoulders. Using the same motions women use to fasten a bra in the back or men use to put a wallet in a back pocket, move your arms in the position shown in Figure 4.10. This exercise is best done standing and is often done in the shower using a washcloth to wash the upper back and a towel to dry it.

Put your head behind your back, then put the other hand behind your back and cross the wrists as shown in the picture. Return the hands to rest at your side.

Repeat this, gradually increasing to five, then more, up to 20 repetitions. Repeat twice daily.

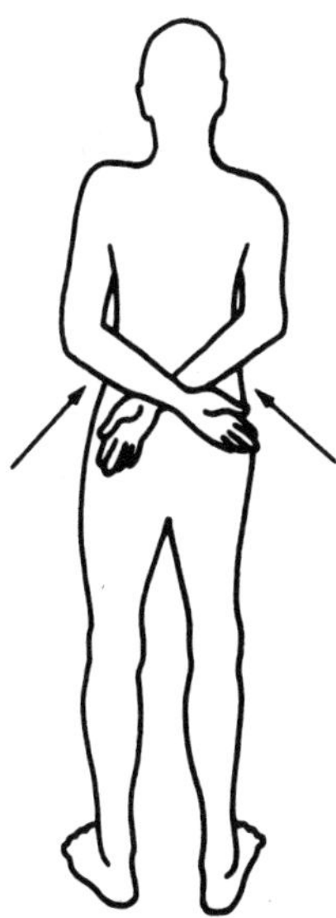

**Figure 4.10.** A shoulder internal rotation exercise.

## Shoulder Flexion

Shoulder flexion begins with holding both arms down at your sides. Raise the left arm straight up and reach overhead toward the ceiling. Now do the same with the right arm. Continue this motion as you alternate left–right–left–right. Repeat this sequence, gradually increasing to five, then more, then up to 20 repetitions, and repeat the exercise twice daily. (See Figure 4.11.)

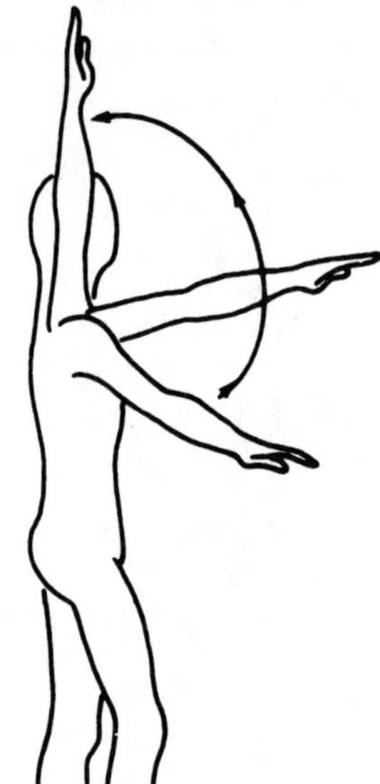

**Figure 4.11.** A shoulder flexion exercise.

## Shoulder Abduction

Shoulder abduction involves raising the arms straight out, away from your side, then raising each arm overhead toward the ceiling and up above your head. Do this with your palm up or palm down.

If this exercise is painful while sitting or standing, do it using a stick (a broom handle will do) while lying on your bed. As you raise your arms, hold the stick with both hands and keep the arms straight, up over your head as far as possible. The strength of the less painful arm will help the painful arm move more easily.

Repeat this exercise, gradually increasing to five, then more, up to 20 repetitions two or three times a day.

This exercise continues as you raise your arms out to the side, one at a time, then slowly make big circles. (See Figure 4.12.)

Repeat this exercise, gradually increasing to five, then more, up to 20 repetitions two or three times a day.

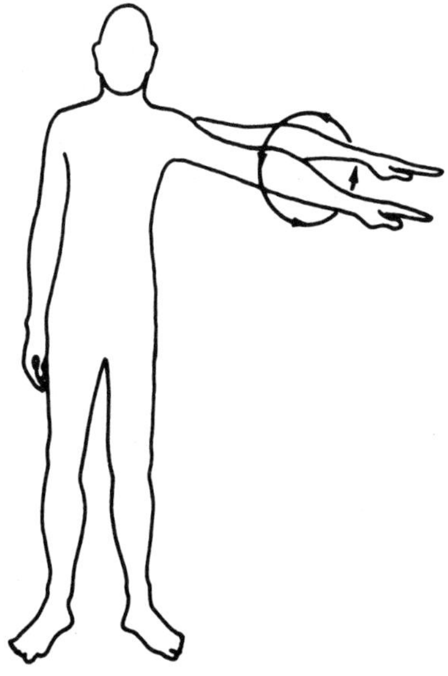

**Figure 4.12.** A shoulder abduction exercise.

## Shoulder Girdle Rotation

This exercise can be done in a sitting or standing position and is fun to do during the day to relieve neck and shoulder tension and maintain shoulder girdle flexibility (see Figure 4.13).

Roll shoulders in a forward circle, raising the shoulders toward the ears in a shrugging motion. Roll shoulders back and chest out as in a military stance. Lower the shoulders and bring the shoulders forward. Think of the movement as a simple shoulder roll in a circle. Now reverse the process, rolling your shoulder girdle in a backward circle.

Repeat this exercise, gradually increasing to five, then more, up to 20 repetitions two or three times a day if possible.

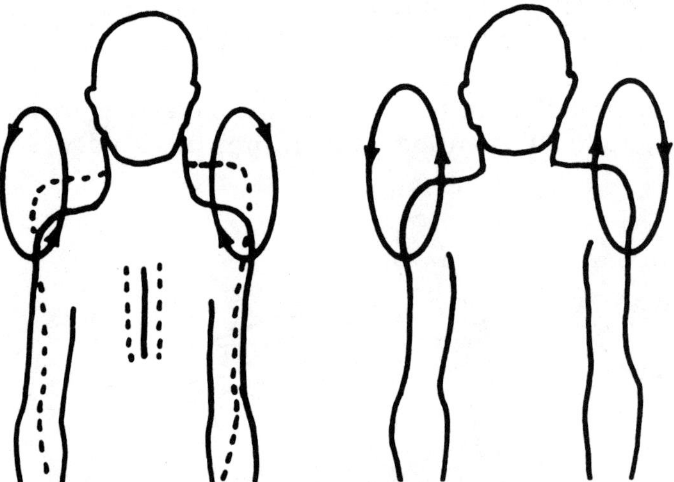

**Figure 4.13.** A shoulder girdle rotation exercise.

## Elbow and Arm Exercises

### Elbow Flexion and Extension

Bend each elbow, bringing the hand toward the top of the shoulder, and then straighten the arm completely, moving it to the side of your body (see Figure 4.14). Be sure to extend the arm fully to the body to gain full motion. Repeat this five times, then more, up to 20 times two or three times each day.

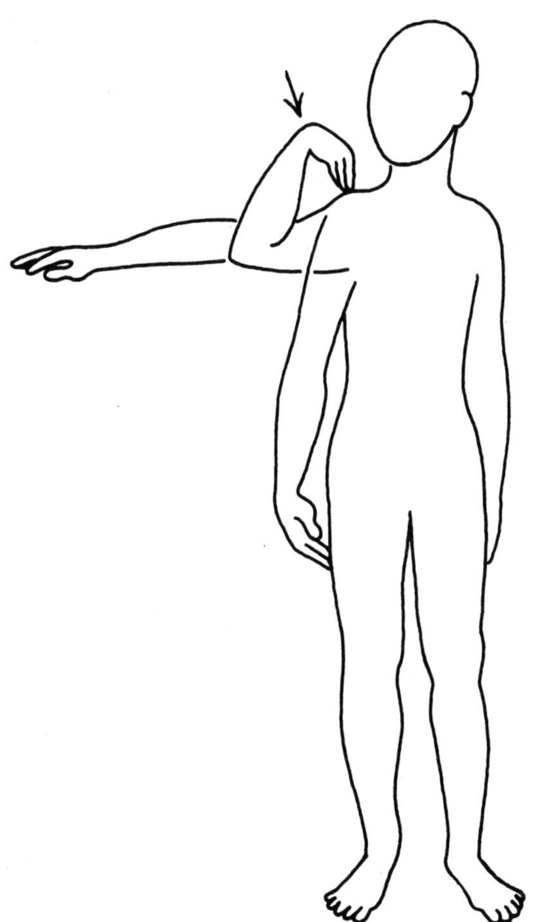

**Figure 4.14.** An elbow flexion and extension exercise.

## Hip Exercises

### Hip Flexion

This is a good exercise sequence to do before you get out of bed in the morning. It will help you limber up for the day. It also stretches the hips, the lower back, and the knees. These exercises can be done on the floor if you are able. (See Figure 4.15.)

Bend each knee toward your chest, one at a time. If you find this difficult, go as far as is comfortable. You can put your hands under a knee and help it bend to the chest. Repeat this, alternating knees. Do five repetitions, then more, up to 20 repetitions two or three times a day if possible.

Now pull both knees to your chest at the same time and hold for six seconds. Gently rock from side to side while holding your knees. Repeat this exercise, increasing gradually to five, then more, up to 20 repetitions a day, if possible.

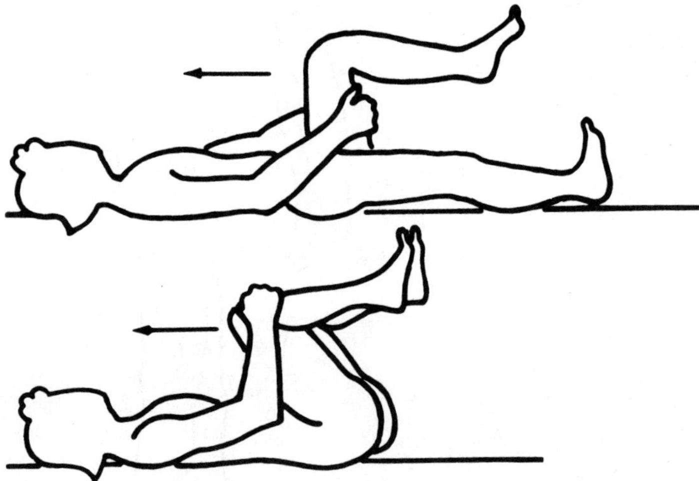

**Figure 4.15.** A hip flexion exercise.

## Hip Abduction

This exercise to improve the mobility of the hips is done lying on your bed or on the floor, whichever is more comfortable for you. (See Figure 4.16.)

Lie on your back. Bend one leg so that your knee is straight up and pointed to the ceiling. Slide the leg out toward the side and then return. Repeat with the opposite leg. Gradually increase to five, then more, up to 20 repetitions two or three times a day if possible.

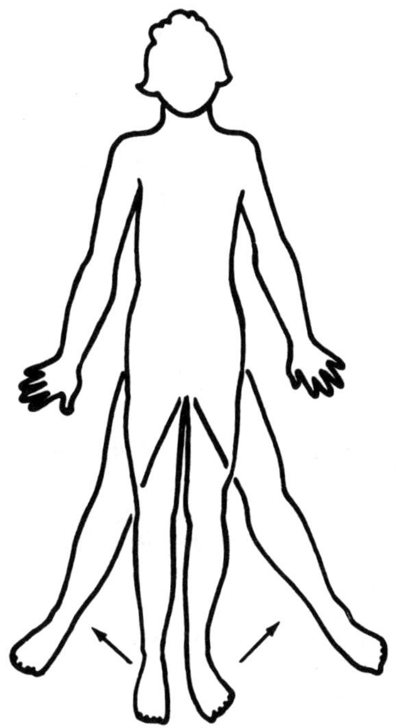

**Figure 4.16.** A hip abduction exercise.

## Hip Extension

For this exercise, lie on your stomach. This can be done on the bed, or on the floor if you are able.

You may want to place a pillow under your stomach to make lying on the floor more comfortable.

With your knee straight, raise either thigh straight up behind you, lifting it several inches off the floor. (See Figure 4.17.) If you lift too far, you will rotate your pelvis and will not get the desired movement. Put this leg down and do the same exercise with the other thigh. When you lift your thigh slightly off the floor, count six seconds while you hold the motion. This is an isometric strengthening exercise to help build muscle strength. You may experience some cramping when you do this exercise because your muscles are working hard to accomplish this motion. Try massaging the cramped muscle. If the cramping persists, talk to your physician or physical therapist.

Repeat this motion and gradually increase up to five, then ten repetitions if you can. Repeat this two times daily if possible.

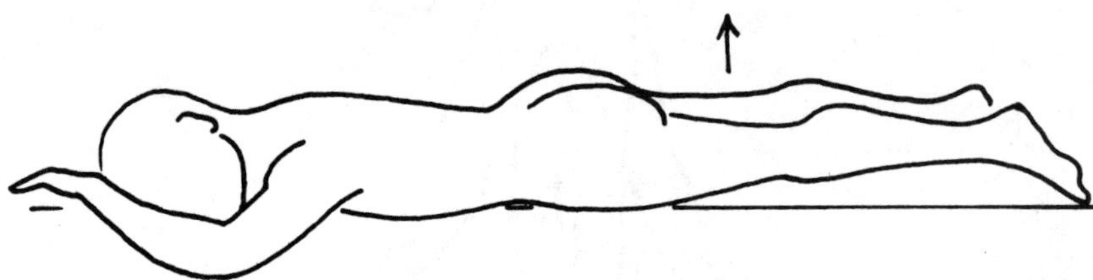

**Figure 4.17.** A hip extension exercise.

## Hip Rotation

To do this exercise, lie on your bed or on the floor. This exercise may seem like a foot exercise but it actually rotates your hips when you keep your legs straight. (See Figure 4.18.)

Lie on your back. Turn your knees in and touch your toes together. Now turn your knees out.

Repeat this exercise, gradually increasing up to five, then more, up to 20 repetitions each session. Repeat this exercise two times daily.

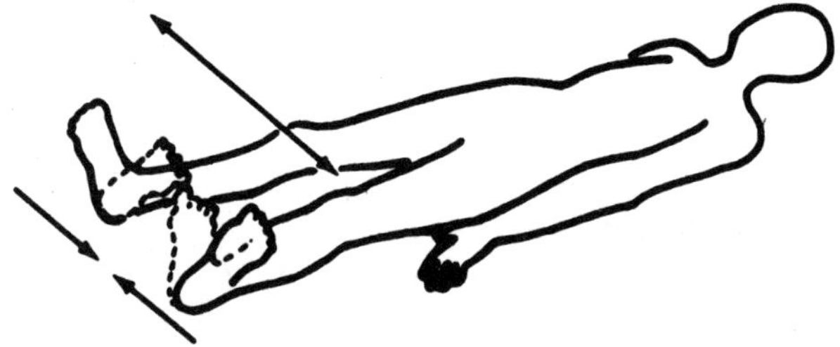

**Figure 4.18.** A hip rotation exercise.

## Knee and Leg Exercises

### Knee Extension and Quad Setting

This is a two-part exercise. Sit in a chair and support your foot on a table or chair that is of comfortable height. (See Figure 4.19.) By simply straightening your leg, you are maintaining knee flexibility. Make the leg as straight as you can tolerate, and hold at that point.

Now, add an isometric strengthening exercise. Try pulling your toes up so the back of the leg is stretched. Tighten your knee cap by pushing the knee down a little, and hold the contraction. You will notice wrinkles in the knee cap, and the muscles in the thigh will tighten. Hold that contraction for six seconds, relax, and repeat. This exercise is especially important for knee stability and standing support. It is called quadriceps muscle (quad) setting. (See Figure 4.19.)

This is a very important exercise to maintain knee strength. Begin gradually and work up to 12 repetitions at one time. Repeat this two or three times a day. This exercise can be done while you relax in a chair watching TV or for a change of position and release of tension at work.

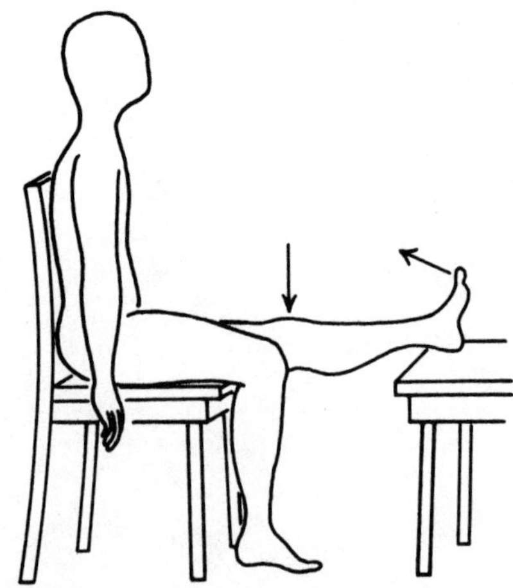

**Figure 4.19.** A knee extension exercise.

Figure 4.20 gives a closer look at how to push the knee down and tighten the knee cap. Hold this position for six counts. This exercise does not require movement of the knee joint. It can be done while in bed, or at other times, without flexion at the knee itself.

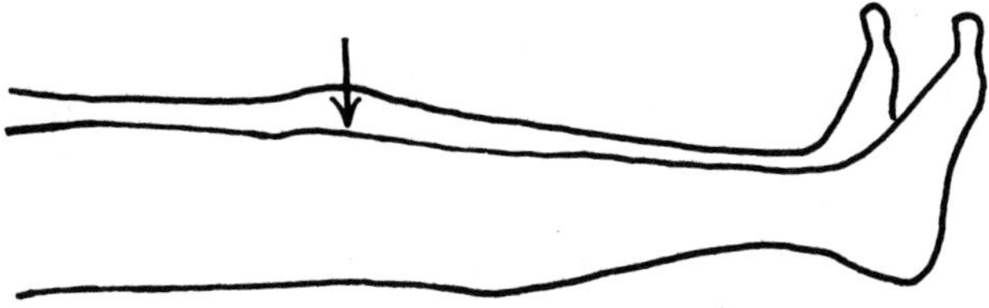

**Figure 4.20.** A quad setting exercise.

## Straight Leg Raise

This exercise helps strengthen the large muscles in the front of the thigh (the quadriceps), which give major support for the knee. It also strengthens the muscles of the abdomen and improves the flexibility of the legs. Do the exercise on your bed or on the floor, whichever is more comfortable for you.

Lie flat on your back. To protect your back during this exercise, you may hug one leg to your chest or simply bend the knee and hip, and rest the foot on the bed or the floor. (See Figure 4.21 for both positions.) Choose the position most comfortable for you. Now, raise the other leg straight up slowly as far as you can, trying to keep the abdomen in and maintaining the back firmly against the floor or bed as in the pelvic tilt–flat back position. When your back begins to arch, stop the raised leg at that point. Hold the position for six seconds. Bend and lower the leg and repeat the exercise. Now do the same for the other leg.

Repeat this exercise, gradually increasing up to five, then more, up to 20 repetitions. If your back hurts or if you have pain in your leg, talk to your physician or physical therapist before you continue.

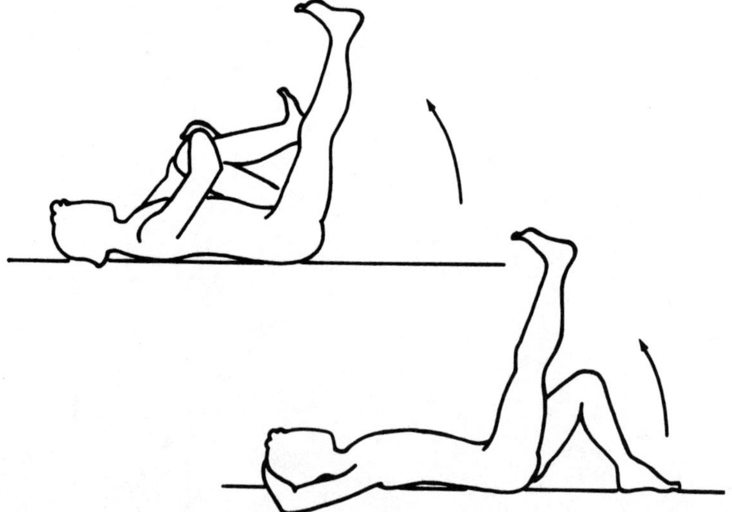

**Figure 4.21.** A straight leg raise exercise.

## Knee Flexion

This exercise can be done on your bed or on the floor, whichever is more comfortable. Lying on your stomach, bend your knee, moving your ankle toward your back as far as you can, then straighten your knee again (see Figure 4.22). Repeat these movements, alternating legs. Gradually increase to five, then more, up to 20 repetitions twice each day.

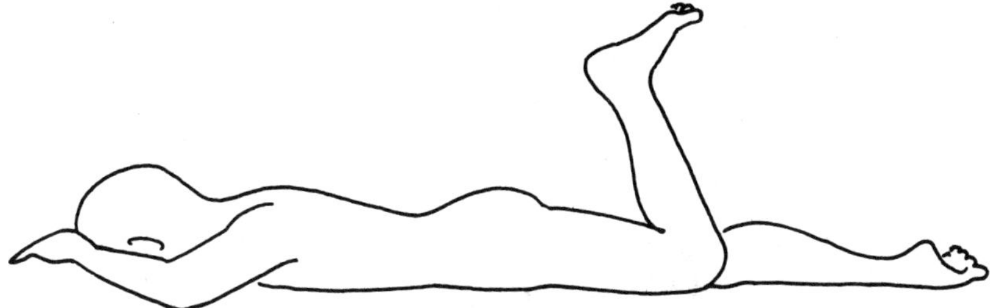

**Figure 4.22.** A knee flexion exercise.

# Ankle and Feet Exercises

## Ankles and Feet

These exercises increase the flexibility and strength in the ankles and feet. If the ankles are stronger and more flexible, they will give better support for the legs and back. The best position for these exercises is sitting in a chair with the feet flat on the floor. (See Figure 4.23.)

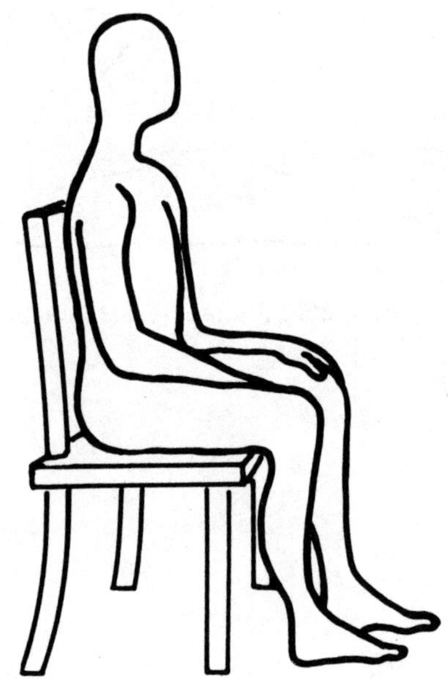

**Figure 4.23.** Position for ankle and foot exercises.

Raise your toes as high as you can while keeping your heel on the floor. (See Figure 4.24.) Then keep your toes down and lift your heels as high as possible.

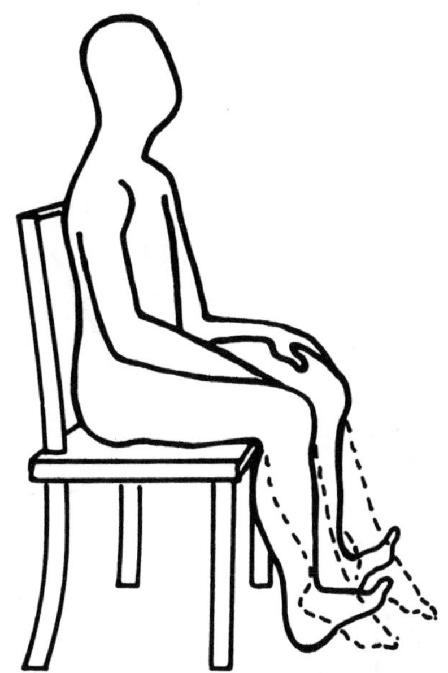

**Figure 4.24.** An ankle and foot exercise.

Lift the inside of each foot and roll the weight over on the outside of the foot. Keep your toes curled down, if possible. The soles of your feet should be turned in facing each other. (See Figure 4.25.)

Rotate the ankle in a circle, curling toes up and down and around in a circle. (See Figure 4.26.)

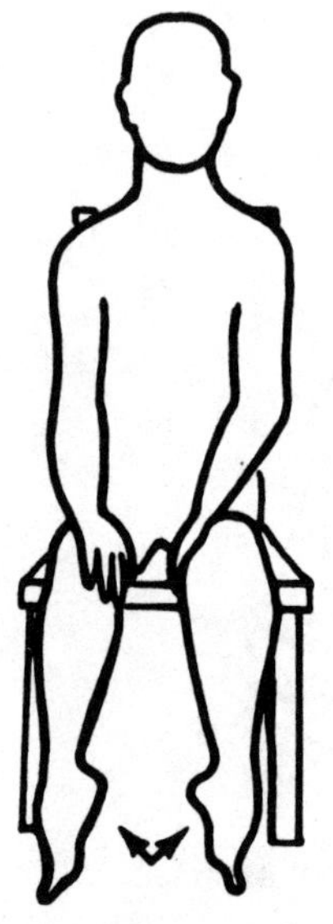

**Figure 4.25.** An ankle and foot exercise.

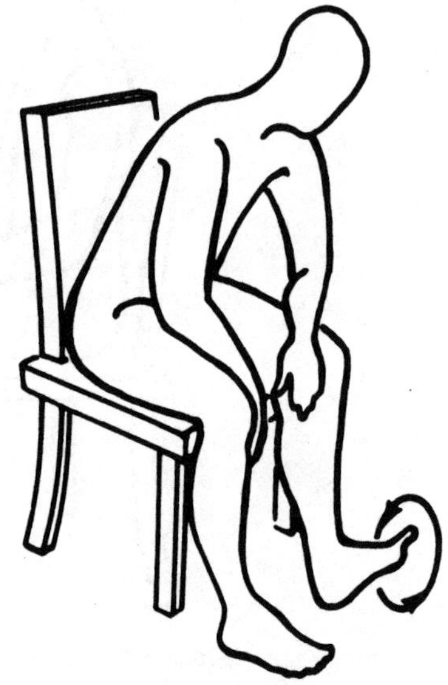

**Figure 4.26.** An ankle and foot exercise.

## Back Exercises

### Cheek-to-Cheek

This is an easy exercise because you can do it anywhere, anytime, and practically in any position. This exercise strengthens the muscles of the buttocks that help support the back and the legs. When sitting, you will actually raise up out of the chair because of the contraction of the muscle groups in the buttocks. (See Figure 4.27.)

Press your buttocks together and hold for a six-second count. Relax and repeat. Gradually increase up to five, then more, up to 20 repetitions. Repeat two times daily.

If you can tolerate this exercise, it can be done frequently during the day, wherever you may be.

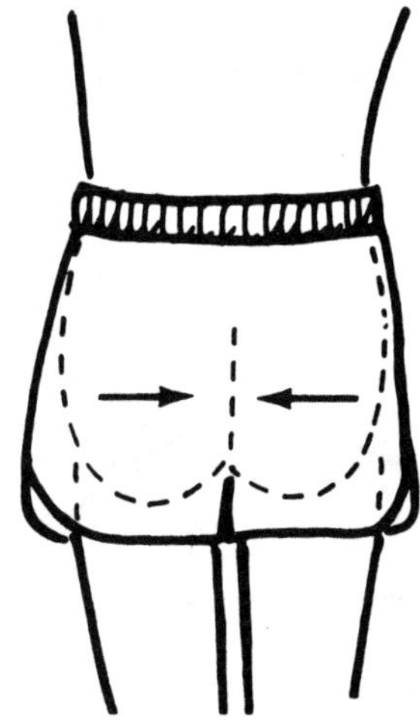

**Figure 4.27.** A cheek-to-cheek exercise.

## Pelvic Tilt

This is one of the best exercises you can do to strengthen your abdominal muscles, which in turn help support your back. This exercise will also help tone your stomach muscles. Do this exercise lying in bed or on the floor, whichever is more comfortable. (See Figure 4.28.)

Relax and raise your arms above your head. Keep your knees bent. Now comes the tricky part: Tighten the muscles of your lower abdomen and your buttocks at the same time, to flatten your back against the floor or bed. This is the flat-back position; hold it for a six-second count. Now relax and repeat.

This is sometimes a difficult exercise to understand. If you have trouble, contact your physical therapist or physician and ask to have the exercise demonstrated.

Repeat this exercise two or three times to start, and work gradually to five, then more, up to 20 repetitions.

This exercise can also be done standing up or sitting in a chair, but these positions probably require some demonstration by a physical therapist.

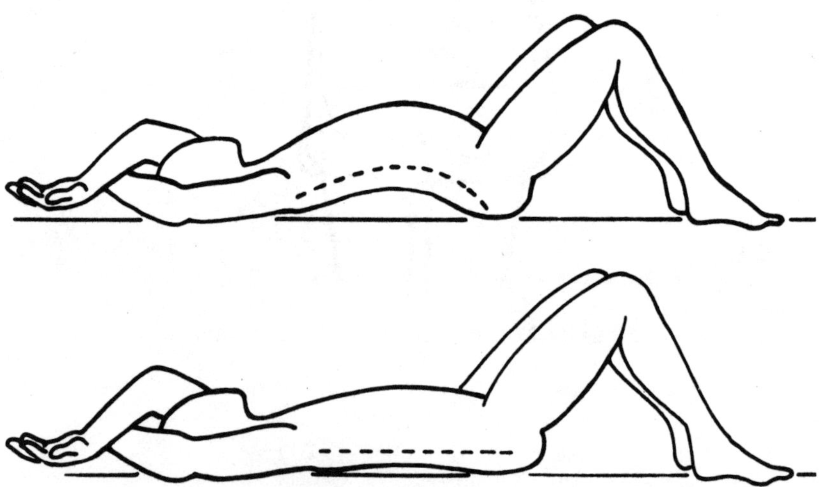

**Figure 4.28.** A pelvic tilt exercise.

## Bridging

This exercise is done lying in bed or on the floor. It strengthens the muscles in the back. (See Figure 4.29.)

Lie on the floor and bend (flex) your hips and knees. Now lift your hips and buttocks off the bed or floor four to six inches, forcing the small of the back out flat; tighten the buttock and hip muscles to maintain this position, and hold it for a count of six seconds. Relax and lower your hips and buttocks to the floor. Repeat.

Repeat this exercise, gradually increasing to five, then more, up to 20 repetitions as tolerated. Repeat this twice daily if possible.

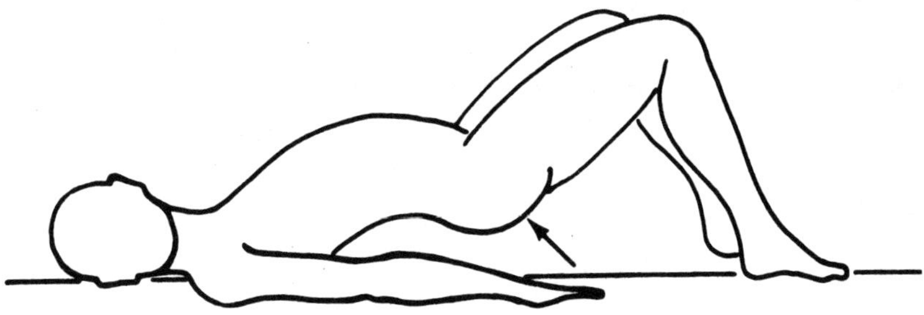

**Figure 4.29.** A bridging exercise.

## Partial Sit-up

This is one of the more vigorous exercises. It is an exercise to build abdominal strength, which in turn better supports the back. (See Figure 4.30.)

To do this exercise, lie on your bed or on the floor, whichever is more comfortable.

Lie on your back with your knees bent. The goals of this exercise are to raise your head and shoulder blades off the floor or bed, then to hold that position for a six-second count. Slowly return to the beginning position of lying on your back. Repeat.

Start this exercise slowly (one or two repetitions) until your body adjusts to the exercise. Gradually increase to five, then ten repetitions. Be sure to do all strengthening exercises and count six seconds aloud. It is very important that you breathe properly while holding this position, and counting aloud will force you to breathe properly. If you experience shortness of breath, stop and talk to your doctor or physical therapist before you resume doing partial sit-ups.

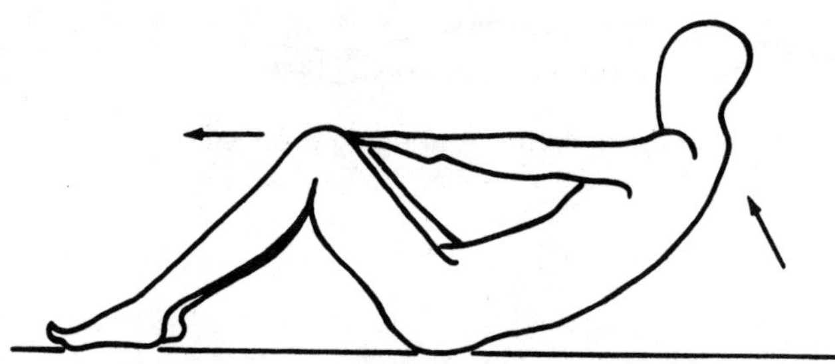

**Figure 4.30.** A partial sit-up exercise.

## Back Extension

This exercise for strengthening the back muscles is to be done while lying on your bed or on the floor in a prone (stomach down) position. (See Figure 4.31.) A pillow may be used under the stomach to help make this position more comfortable.

Raise your head, arms, and legs off the floor. Do not bend your knees. Keep your body straight in extension. Hold for several seconds while you count aloud. Relax and repeat.

Gradually increase this exercise up to five, then ten repetitions. If you experience discomfort, check with your physician or physical therapist before you continue.

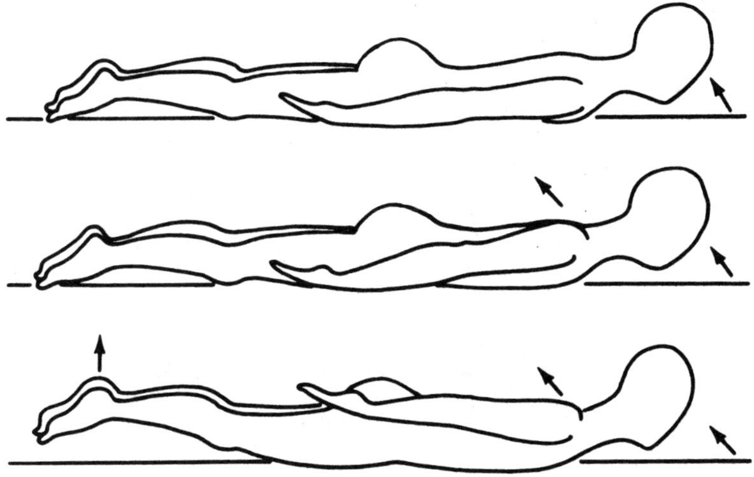

**Figure 4.31.** A back extension exercise.

## Cat Camel

Do not do this exercise for strengthening the back muscles if you have very painful knees, ankles, or hands. It places pressure on these areas. (See Figure 4.32.)

The position for this exercise is a crawling position. Your hands must be directly under your shoulders. Take a deep breath and arch your back as a frightened cat does, lowering your head. Hold that position while you count the six seconds aloud. Now exhale and drop the arched back slowly, raising your head.

Start this exercise slowly with one or two repetitions. Increase up to five and then ten repetitions if possible.

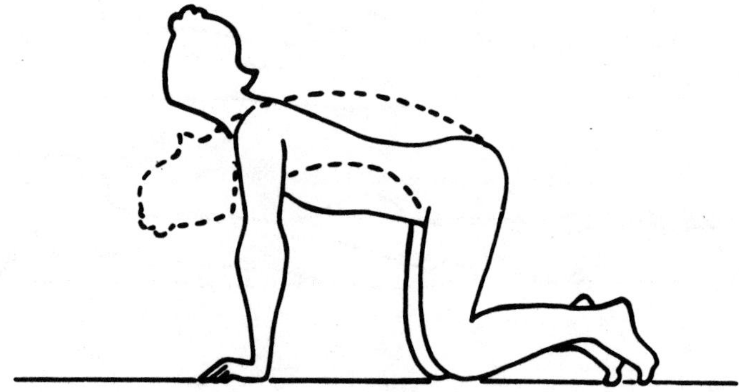

**Figure 4.32.** A cat camel exercise.

## Wall Push

This exercise is good for the back because it encourages the body extension positions.

Stand spread-eagled against a solid wall. Now arch your back inward slowly.

Repeat this exercise and gradually increase repetitions from one to five or more. This exercise is fun because you can do it any time you feel you need a good body stretch. Repeat two times daily. (See Figure 4.33.)

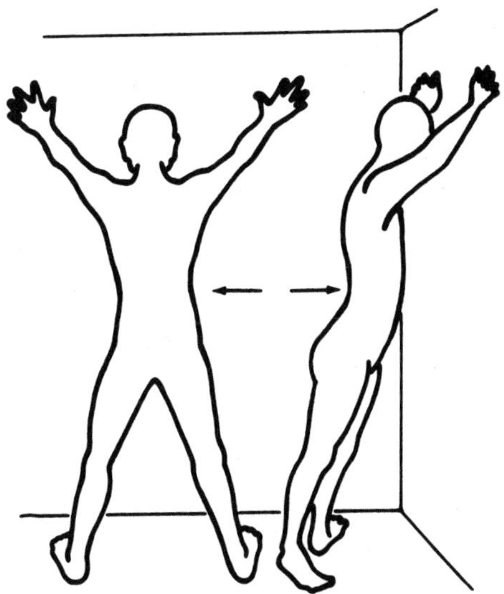

**Figure 4.33.** Wall push.

## Back Flexibility

Lie on your back on the floor with your knees bent and your feet flat on the floor. Raise your hands toward the ceiling. Now move your arms and turn your head to the right, while your knees move to the left. (See Figure 4.34.) Reverse the above, then repeat. Gradually increase up to five and then ten repetitions daily.

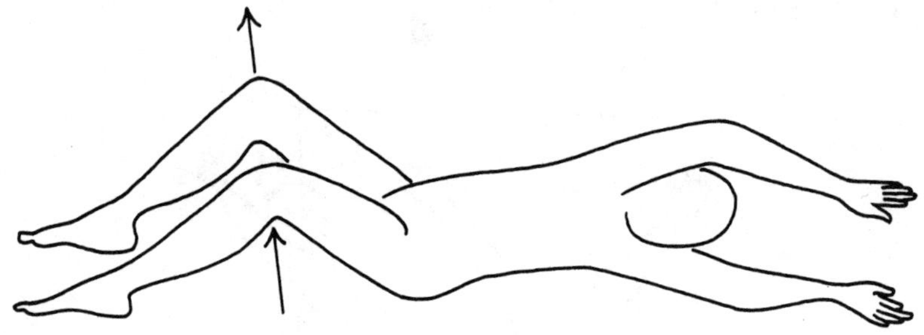

**Figure 4.34.** A back flexibility exercise.

## Bicycling

Lying on your back, move your feet and legs in the air as if you were riding a bicycle. (See Figure 4.35.) Count to six, and relax. Repeat, then gradually increase to five and then ten repetitions once or twice daily if tolerable.

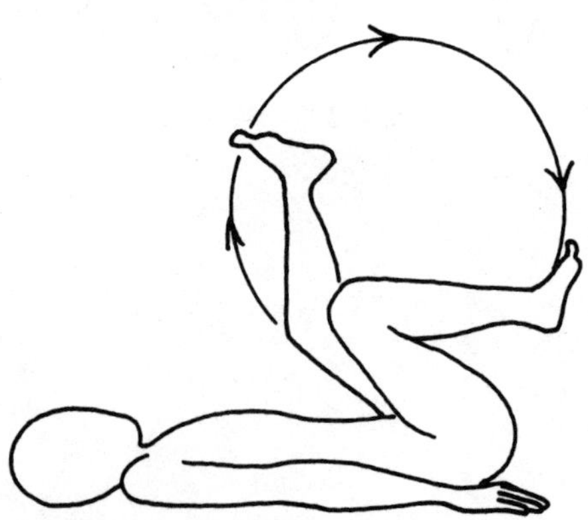

**Figure 4.35.** A bicycling exercise.

## Chest and Posture Exercises

### Deep Breathing

This exercise improves the movement of the chest and helps your posture. Perform this exercise in the rest position, with your hands comfortably placed behind your head. You will also do a good shoulder rotation exercise by placing your hands behind your head. This position allows your rib cage and chest to expand fully. Bend your knees to protect your back. (See Figure 4.36.)

Once you are in this comfortable position, breathe deeply and raise your chest while filling your lungs completely. Hold for about two seconds and then exhale by drawing your upper abdomen in. Take the next breath against the uplifted chest. This may be a difficult exercise to understand without a demonstration. Contact your physical therapist or physician for assistance.

Being this exercise slowly and gradually increase the repetitions from five on up to 20.

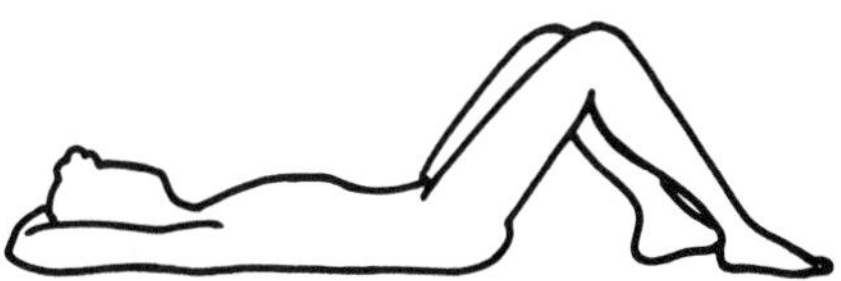

**Figure 4.36.** A deep breathing exercise.

## Wing Back

This is another exercise that is good for the back because it encourages backward bending of the arms and body. (See Figure 4.37.)

Do this exercise in a relaxed standing position. Lift your elbows to shoulder height with the arms bent. Now straighten the arms backward. Hold.

Repeat this exercise and gradually increase the repetitions. Start with five and work up to ten, then 20 as tolerated. Repeat the exercise two times daily.

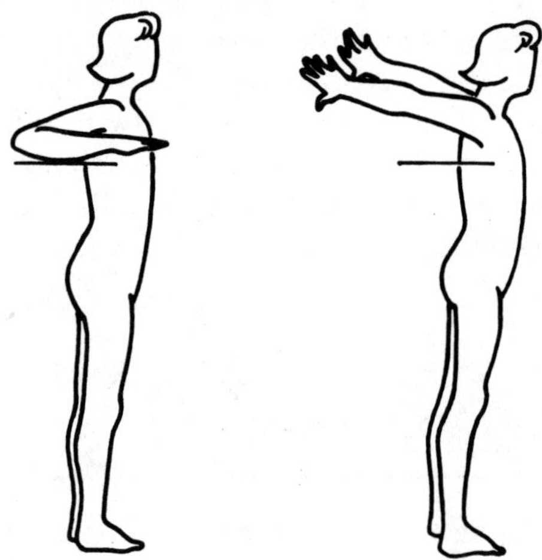

**Figure 4.37.** A wing back exercise.

## Arm Swing

Posture is important when doing these exercises. Their objective is to emphasize extension of the back and neck and increased expansion of the chest. Stand comfortably with your knees, back, and shoulders slightly relaxed. (See Figure 4.38.)

Start with your hands down and crossed in front of you. Swing them slowly up and out over the head, reaching back as far as you can. When your arms are up, take a deep breath. When you lower your arms, exhale. Repeat.

Repeat this exercise, gradually increasing up to five, then ten repetitions. This exercise should be repeated two times daily.

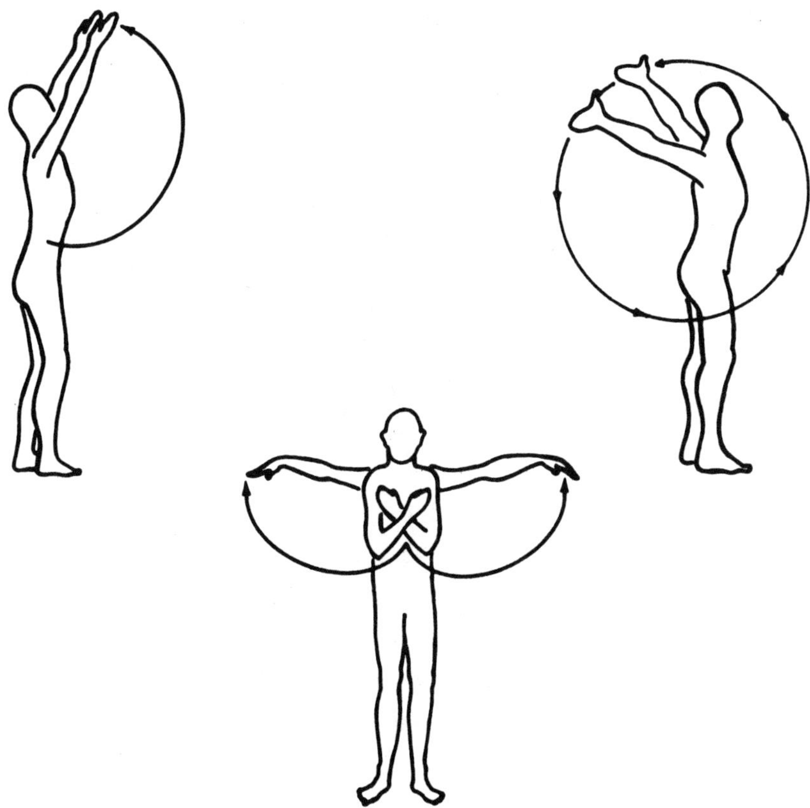

**Figure 4.38.** An arm swing exercise.

## Diagonal Arm Swing

Start with both arms out to the side at hip height. Move your hand diagonally across your body and upward over your head. Twisting the trunk, turn the head to watch the hand, inhale on the upswing, and exhale on the downswing. Reverse and do the other side. Repeat. Gradually increase up to five, then ten repetitions daily. (See Figure 4.39.)

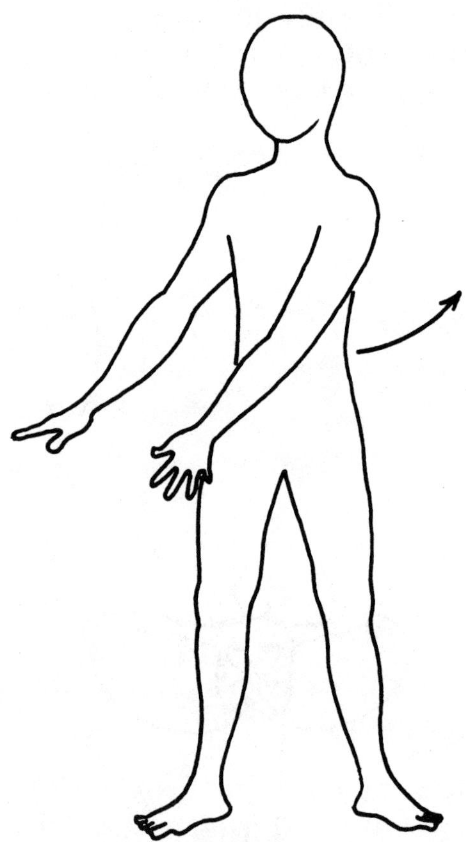

**Figure 4.39.** A diagonal arm swing exercise.

## Strengthening Exercises

When the above exercises can be easily performed up to 20 or more repetitions without pain or other discomfort, it may be possible to begin a more aggressive type of exercise in order to gain more muscle strength. Before you attempt strengthening exercises, discuss them with your physician or physical therapist to be sure that they are safe for you.

Two easy ways to begin to build more muscle strength are by using (1) isometric exercises and (2) light weights.

Isometric exercises use muscle contractions without joint movement. The resistance should be very light at first, then increased very gradually as pain allows and as strength increases.

This section gives a few examples of isometric exercises that use a rubber or elastic band, or the hands, as resistance.

Light hand or ankle weights may sometimes be used to strengthen muscles. The exercises described here can be performed with the addition of one- or two-pound weights on the ankles, feet, arms, or hands. Weights must be very light (not exceeding two pounds) to avoid adding excess stress to the joints being exercised.

The light weights can be strapped to the hand, wrist, or ankle. If no weights are available, we suggest holding canned goods in the hands to exercise the shoulders and elbows as tolerated. A sock filled with sand and tied at the top can be used as a weight for the wrist or ankle in some exercises.

Remember, it is more important to begin an exercise program gradually and safely than to do a large amount of exercise quickly. Your exercise program should be part of a long-term plan using the *basic treatment program.* Stay with it, and you'll be surprised how quickly you can do many more exercises than you expected. After a few weeks to a few months, you will begin to feel more flexibility and more strength, and you will have less pain in the joints and much more activity. You will be able to do the things you could not do earlier because of pain and stiffness.

## Isometric Exercises for the Neck

With one hand or forearm placed on the forehead, move the head so that you can look directly downward. At the same time, resist this movement with the hand or forearm. Hold for five to six seconds. Breathe, then repeat. Gradually increase up to five, then ten times twice each day.

Now, with the hand or forearm on the back of the head, try to look upward while resisting the movement with the hand or forearm, as shown in Figure 4.40. Hold for five to six seconds. Breathe, then repeat. Gradually increase up to five, then ten times twice a day.

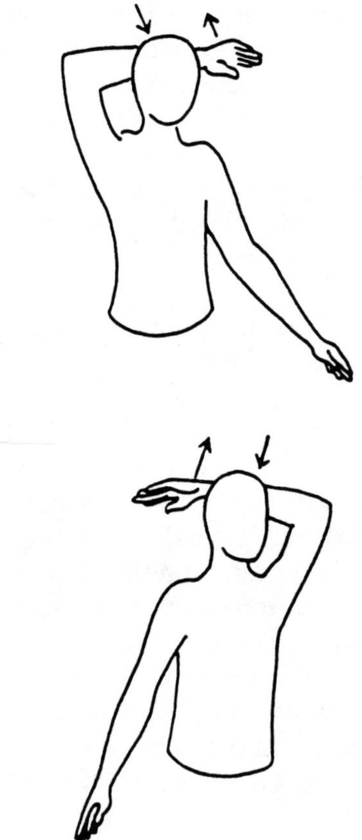

**Figure 4.40.** Isometric exercises for the neck.

## Isometric Exercises for the Shoulders

Using a rubber or elastic band (your physician or physical therapist can supply this), pull both arms out toward the side of the body as shown. When the band is tight, giving resistance, hold in that position for five to six seconds. (See Figure 4.41.)

Pull one arm upward and the opposite arm downward. When the band is tight, giving resistance, hold in that position for five to six seconds.

With one arm behind the back and the other arm behind the head, pull upward and downward, as shown, until the band is tight and gives resistance. Hold for five to six seconds.

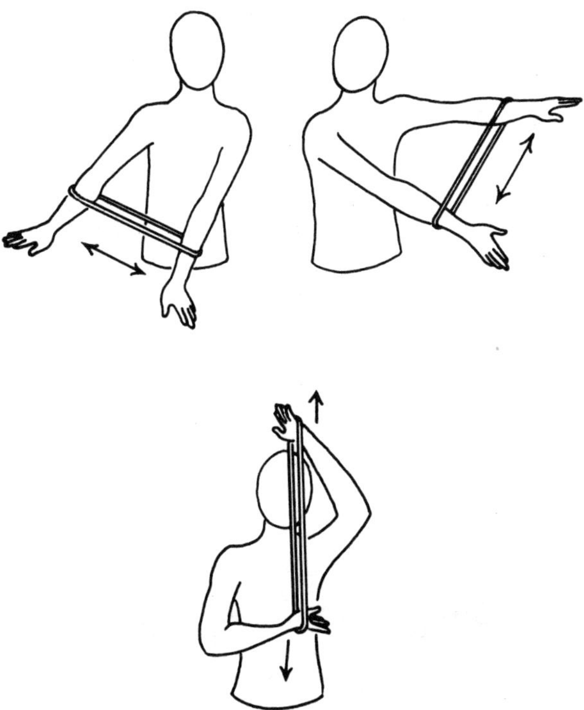

**Figure 4.41.** Isometric exercises for the shoulders.

## Isometric Exercises for the Elbows

With the elbows bent and the elastic band placed around the forearms, try to bend one elbow toward your chest while straightening the other elbow out. (See Figure 4.42.) Hold for five to six seconds when the band becomes tight. The band should be 12 to 18 inches in length. Your physical therapist or physician can help if you have questions about these exercises.

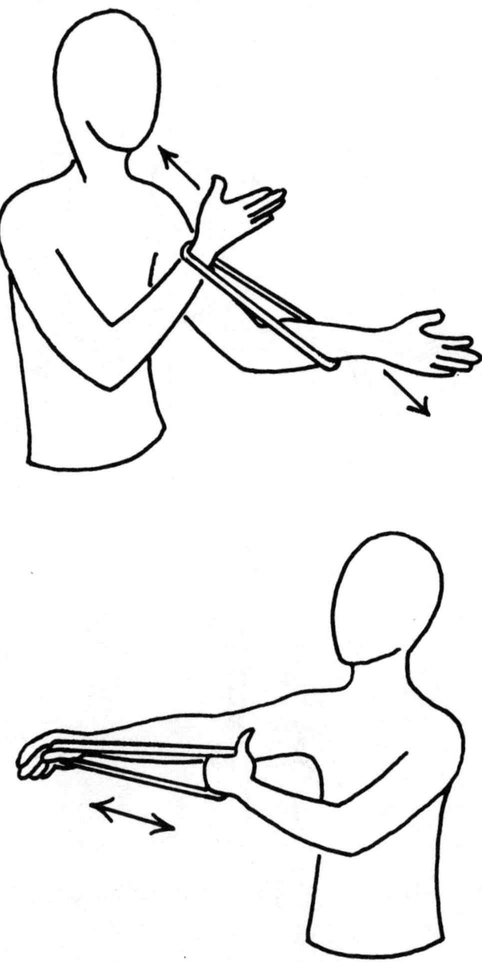

**Figure 4.42.** An isometric exercise for the elbows.

## Isometric Exercises for the Hips

Sitting in a chair with the hands on your outer thighs, pull your legs apart while both hands push inward (see Figure 4.43). The push gives resistance to the movement. Hold five or six seconds. Do once, then twice, then gradually increase, as you can, up to ten times twice daily.

This exercise can also be done with the hands on the inside of the thighs. The legs then pull together while the hands push outward.

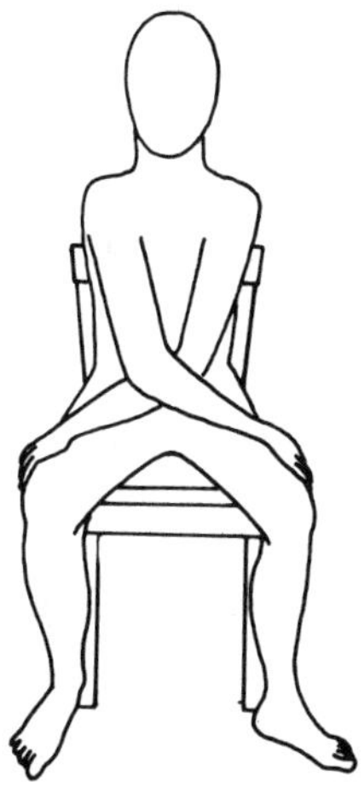

**Figure 4.43.** An isometric exercise for the hips.

Place the elastic band above the ankles. Lying face-down on the bed or floor, raise one leg upward while the other leg remains on the bed or floor (see Figure 4.44). Hold for five or six seconds. Repeat once, then twice, then gradually increase up to ten times twice daily.

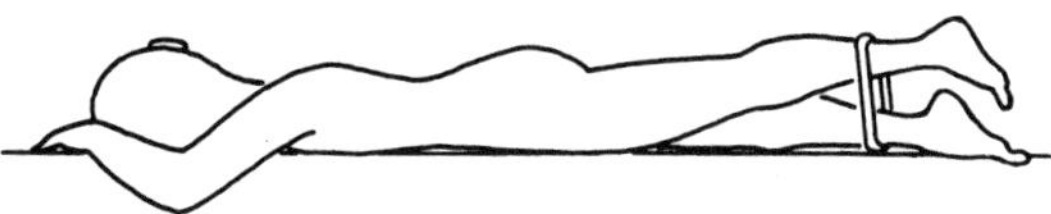

**Figure 4.44.** An isometric exercise for the hips.

Stand up straight and raise up on the toes. Hold this position for five to six seconds, then reverse the weight onto the heels (see Figure 4.45). Repeat once, then twice, then gradually increase up to ten times twice daily. This can help strengthen the ankles and the calf muscles.

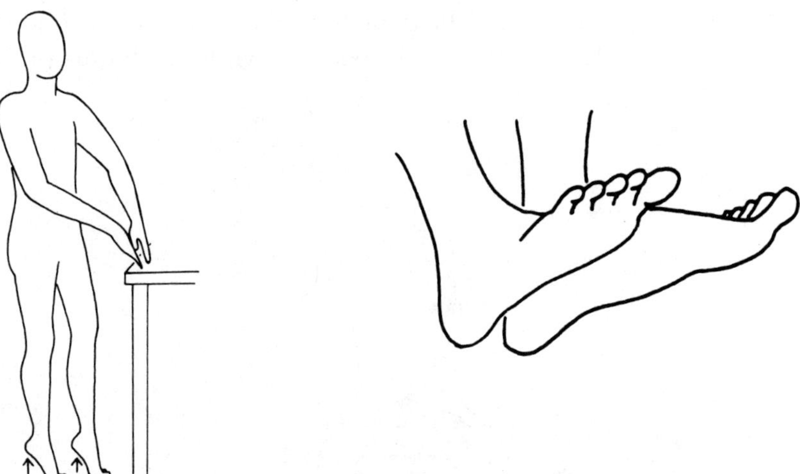

**Figure 4.45.** Isometric exercises for the hips.

## Examples of Exercises Using Light Weights

Sitting in a chair, with the weight strapped at the ankle, straighten the knee out and lower it back down to the floor. Be sure to go only as far as is comfortable, and use only one-pound weights. Repeat once, then twice, and then gradually increase up to five or ten times twice daily if you can do this without pain (see Figure 4.46 and 4.47).

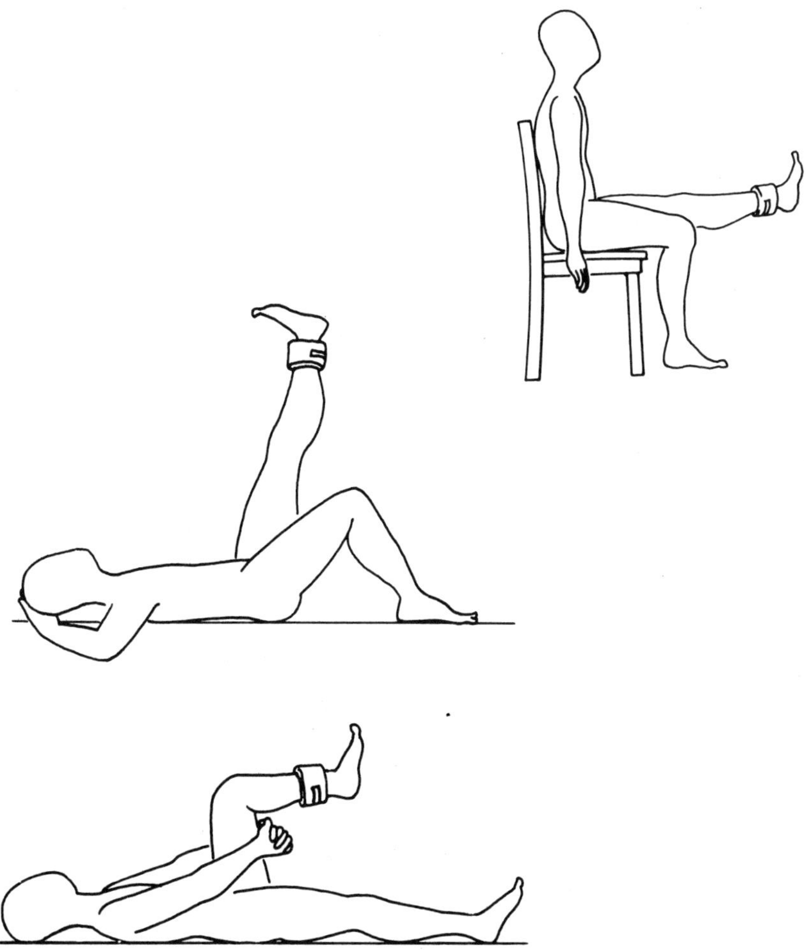

**Figure 4.46.** Examples of isometric exercises using light weights.

With a weight strapped around the wrist, raise the arm upward toward the head and then back to the side of the body. Repeat once, then twice, then gradually increase up to ten times twice daily.

Arm circles can be done with the weights around the wrist. Start with a small circle, then gradually increase the size of the circle. Repeat once, then twice, then gradually increase up to ten times twice each day, if possible. Don't overdo this exercise at first, and remember to use a light weight (one pound) at first.

Lying on the bed, slide one leg out to the side and back to the middle with the weight strapped just above the ankle. Do this for both legs. Repeat once, then twice, then gradually increase up to ten times twice each day as long as you can comfortably do the repetitions without pain.

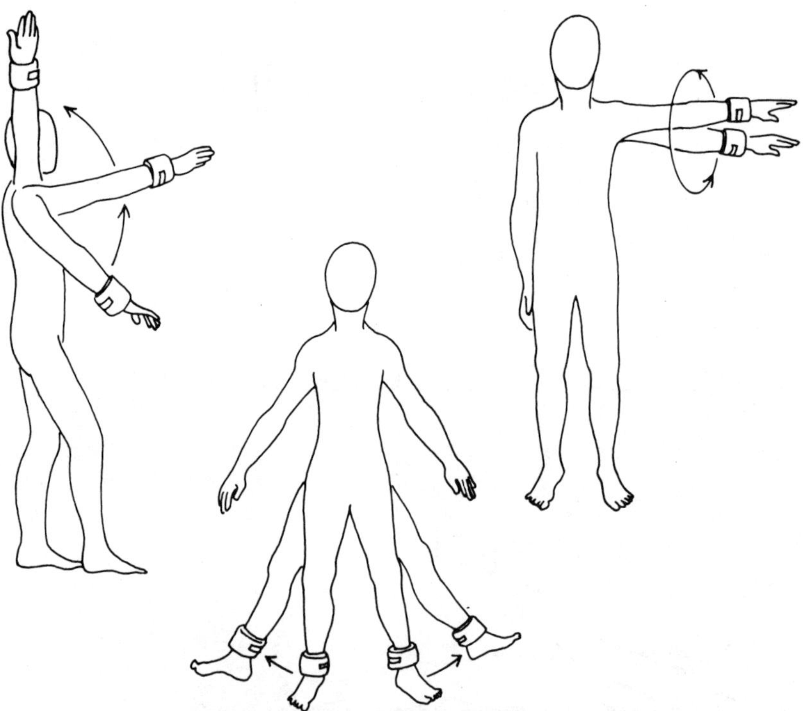

**Figure 4.47.** Examples of isometric exercises using light weights.

CHAPTER FIVE

# Preventing Further Back Pain

People with back pain frequently ask, "Once the pain is gone or much improved after one or two weeks, can anything be done to prevent the attacks?" Although the causes of the most common type of acute back pain are not known, and there is no absolute cure, there are steps you can take to make the attacks come less often, last a shorter time, and be less severe.

The prevention measures described in this book do not require a drastic life-style change. Most people are able to incorporate the program of exercise, weight control, body conditioning, and proper diet into their daily schedules without much difficulty. Most of our patients report that these measures intended to prevent their back pain actually enhance their overall well-being. They feel stronger, look healthier, and have more energy.

## Don't Stop the Exercises

When the pain improves, don't stop the exercise program. Remember that it takes weeks to months to build stronger muscles. You can make your back muscles stronger and more flexible, but it takes time. The exercise program outlined in this book may be the most important step available to you for prevention of future back pain.

Remember how painful the back pain was. Remind yourself that a regular back exercise program can help decrease the chance of that pain returning.

Finding the time to do the exercises may seem more difficult than performing them, but once you learn the exercises and their sequence becomes routine, you will be surprised to see that they can be done in a few minutes each day. Some of our patients tell us that they "can do without" the exercises because they are active during the day at work and other activities. There is a difference between activity and exercise. It is no coincidence that our busiest patients are also those with the worst back pain. In most cases, daily activities do not strengthen the back muscles and may actually increase the stress on them and the amount of work they must perform. For example, sitting at a desk and leaning slightly forward puts a large amount of constant pressure on the bones and discs of the lower back, creating more stress on the back muscles.

There is no replacement for making your back muscles stronger and more flexible. You might find the time for exercises by awakening a few minutes early, or doing the exercises at the end of your evening, or setting aside a few minutes during the day. Some people prefer to do all the exercises at one session each day, rather than twice daily. The important point is to do them regularly.

Our patients find that the exercises become much easier after a few weeks, and the results they see even in that short time make the effort worthwhile. *Find a way* to insert the exercises into your daily routine. Once you maintain a regular program for a few months, it will become unnatural *not* to do them.

## Control Your Weight

Extra body weight puts additional stress on the spine, the muscles, and the other soft tissues in the back. It makes sense

## Table 5.1
## Metropolitan Height and Weight

### MEN

| Height Feet | Height Inches | Small Frame | Medium Frame | Large Frame |
|---|---|---|---|---|
| 5 | 2 | 128–134 | 131–141 | 138–150 |
| 5 | 3 | 130–136 | 133–143 | 140–153 |
| 5 | 4 | 132–138 | 135–145 | 142–156 |
| 5 | 5 | 134–140 | 137–148 | 144–160 |
| 5 | 6 | 136–142 | 139–151 | 146–164 |
| 5 | 7 | 138–145 | 142–154 | 149–168 |
| 5 | 8 | 140–148 | 145–157 | 152–172 |
| 5 | 9 | 142–151 | 148–160 | 155–176 |
| 5 | 10 | 144–154 | 151–163 | 158–180 |
| 5 | 11 | 146–157 | 154–166 | 161–184 |
| 6 | 0 | 149–160 | 157–170 | 164–188 |
| 6 | 1 | 152–164 | 160–174 | 168–192 |
| 6 | 2 | 155–168 | 164–178 | 172–197 |
| 6 | 3 | 158–172 | 167–182 | 176–202 |
| 6 | 4 | 162–176 | 171-187 | 181-207 |

Weights at Ages 25–59 Based on Lowest Mortality. Weight in Pounds According to Frame (in indoor clothing weighing 5 lbs., shoes with 1″ heels).

### WOMEN

| Height Feet | Height Inches | Small Frame | Medium Frame | Large Frame |
|---|---|---|---|---|
| 4 | 10 | 102–111 | 109–121 | 118–131 |
| 4 | 11 | 103–113 | 111–123 | 120–134 |
| 5 | 0 | 104–115 | 113–126 | 122–137 |
| 5 | 1 | 106–118 | 115–129 | 125–140 |
| 5 | 2 | 108–121 | 118–132 | 128–143 |
| 5 | 3 | 111–124 | 121–135 | 131–147 |
| 5 | 4 | 114–127 | 124–138 | 134–151 |
| 5 | 5 | 117–130 | 127–141 | 137–155 |
| 5 | 6 | 120–133 | 130–144 | 140–159 |
| 5 | 7 | 123–136 | 133–147 | 143–163 |
| 5 | 8 | 126–139 | 136–150 | 146–167 |
| 5 | 9 | 129–142 | 139–153 | 149–170 |
| 5 | 10 | 132–145 | 142–156 | 152–173 |
| 5 | 11 | 135–148 | 145–159 | 155–176 |
| 6 | 0 | 138–151 | 148–162 | 158–179 |

Weights at Ages 25–59 Based on Lowest Mortality. Weight in Pounds According to Frame (in indoor clothing weighing 3 lbs., shoes with 1″ heels).

Source of basic data: *1979 Build Study,* Society of Actuaries and Association of Life Insurance Medical Directors of America, 1980. Reprinted with permission from Metropolitan Life Insurance Company, New York, New York.

that losing your extra pounds would lower the work load on your back. You don't have to be at your exact ideal body weight as stated in Table 5.1, but the closer you can get, the better your back should respond.

If you are overweight, begin a slow but steady weight loss program as detailed in Chapter Six. A loss of only one pound a week is an excellent goal. This rate of weight loss may not sound fast enough, but it adds up to 52 pounds in one year. If you lose at this slow and steady rate, your chances of keeping the weight off are much higher.

## Add a Conditioning Exercise

The easiest way to do a conditioning exercise is to add a simple walking program to your daily schedule. Pick a short distance and walk it daily. You may be able to set a regular time for your walking each day, or, if necessary, move the time around according to your schedule. Just be sure that you gradually increase the distance you walk daily. You will be surprised at how quickly you'll be able to see progress.

Whatever conditioning exercise you choose, it should be convenient and one you don't mind doing. If you don't enjoy walking, try bicycle riding, an exercise bike, swimming, or some other exercise you enjoy. Many of our patients prefer to have an exercise bike or treadmill in their home so that they can exercise anytime, day or night, at their convenience. There is no threat to safety, no problem from bad weather, and no excuse for not exercising when the equipment is available at home.

## Protect the Back

While you're working at strengthening your back and removing the stress of extra weight, you can protect your back by being smart during daily activities. The simple tips in the following sections can help you decrease the amount of work needed and the force put on your back. The reasoning makes sense: If your back is stronger and is given less unusual stress, you may have less back pain.

Start by looking at your daily routine activities.

## Sitting

Did you know that, at many times each day, the discs in the lower back endure pressures three or four times the body weight? For example, when you are sitting and have no back support, the pressure on the lower back is about 40 percent higher than when you are standing! The pressure is even higher when you are sitting and leaning slightly forward. Think of the number of times—or hours—you do this each day.

There are some simple ways to decrease the force that the discs in your back must bear. For example, having a backrest on your chair, or resting your lower back against the back of the chair, or using a support for the lower back all decrease the pressure. Using armrests also helps ease the back pressure. Some car makers now build a lumbar support into the driver's seat of their cars, to help decrease pressure on the back during long rides.

Try to choose a chair that gives firm support, allows your back to be fairly straight, and gives good lower back support. Your feet should comfortably reach the floor—a most necessary factor in the chair you use at work or other common activities. Improper position while sitting can be a major cause of strain on the back. (See Fig. 5.1(a) and Fig. 5.1(b).)

If your job involves sitting at a desk for long periods of time, stand up for a few minutes every hour or two to stretch backward or walk.

Be careful of the height of the desk at which you work. If the level of your work is uncomfortably high or low, the pressures on your spine from the lower back to the neck will be increased. You may need to adjust the height of the work or trade for another desk to make this height more comfortable.

Sitting properly can cause less pain in the back. Try to sit in a firm chair, with your buttocks against the back of the chair, your feet comfortably flat on the floor, and your back not bent over. Armrests can result in less pressure and pain in the back.

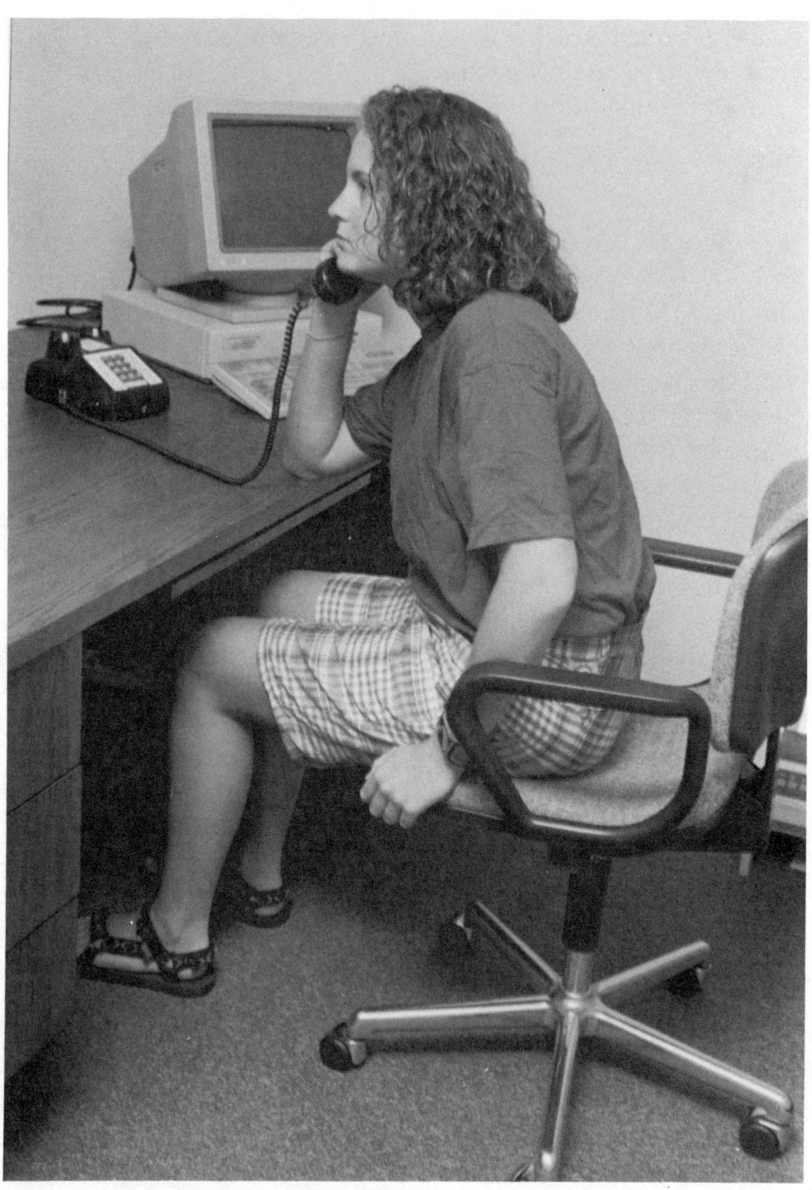

**Figure 5.1(a).** Poor posture can aggravate back pain.

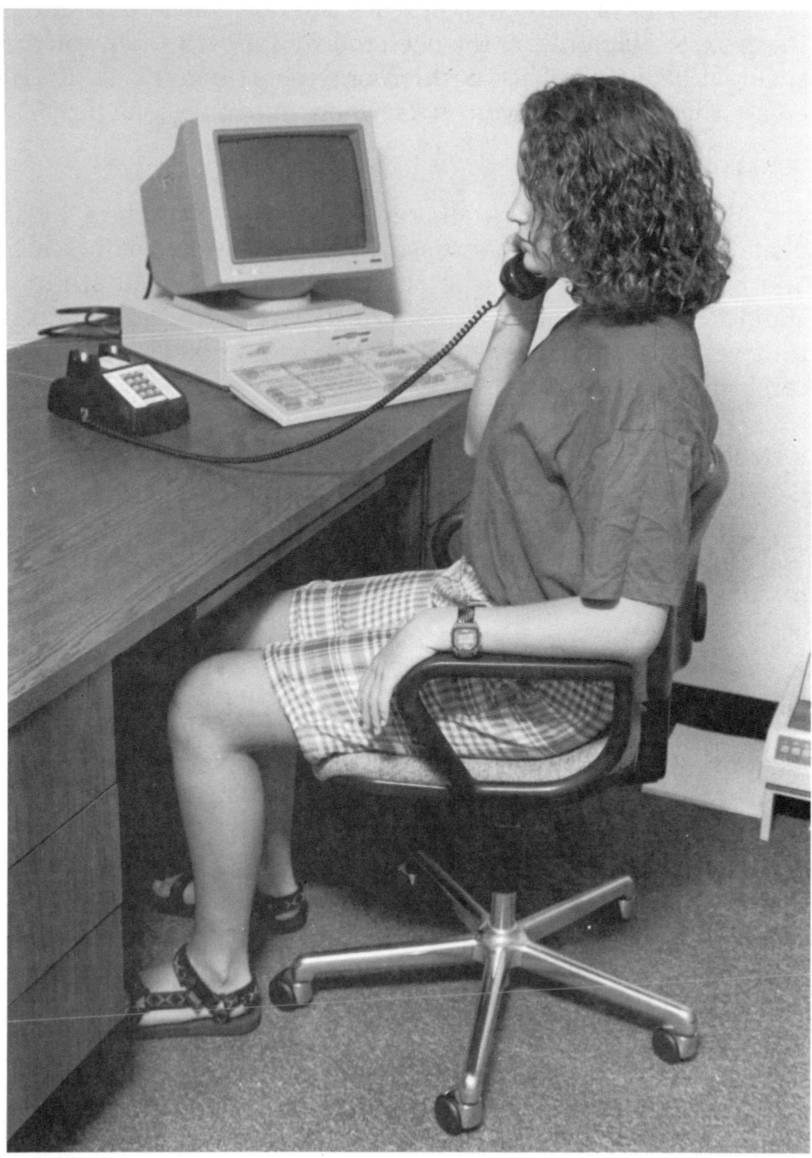

**Figure 5.1(b).** Sitting improperly can cause pain in the back. Try to sit in a firm chair, buttocks against the back of the chair, with feet comfortably flat on the floor and back not bent over. Armrests can also ease pressure and pain in the back.

The arms of your chair at work should be able to go under the desk, to help prevent the need to lean forward when you are sitting. Use a lower back cushion or support if you need to decrease the pressure on your back when you sit for long periods.

## Standing

When you stand or walk, remember that when the spine is bent over even a little, the pressures on the lower back increase. You place the least pressure on your back when you are in a standing position with your back fairly straight. You don't need to have perfect posture, but thinking about your back a little can bring great rewards.

If your daily activity involves much standing, wear comfortable shoes that have good support. Try to avoid higher heels. A lightweight athletic shoe is a good choice.

Avoid standing in one position for long periods at a time. You might try placing a rubber mat in the area if you must stand for long periods. The mat will give some cushioning to your feet and back.

When you stand, you can occasionally rest or "prop" one foot on a box or stool for comfort. (See Figure 5.2.)

Hold your abdominal muscles in. Avoid the "swayback" position, which puts higher pressures on the back.

## Sleeping

Use a firm mattress on your bed for good support. If your mattress is too soft, it may put extra stress on your back. Remember that mattresses don't last forever. If your mattress is more than five years old, it may need to be replaced. Some people find the most relief for back pain when they sleep on a water bed.

For sleeping, choose the position that is most comfortable. If your neck or upper back is painful, pillows made to fit the contour of the neck are available. You may want to try one of these, although their results for relief of pain vary with individuals.

For people who have arthritis in the back, it is usually a good idea to try to spend some part of the sleep hours lying on

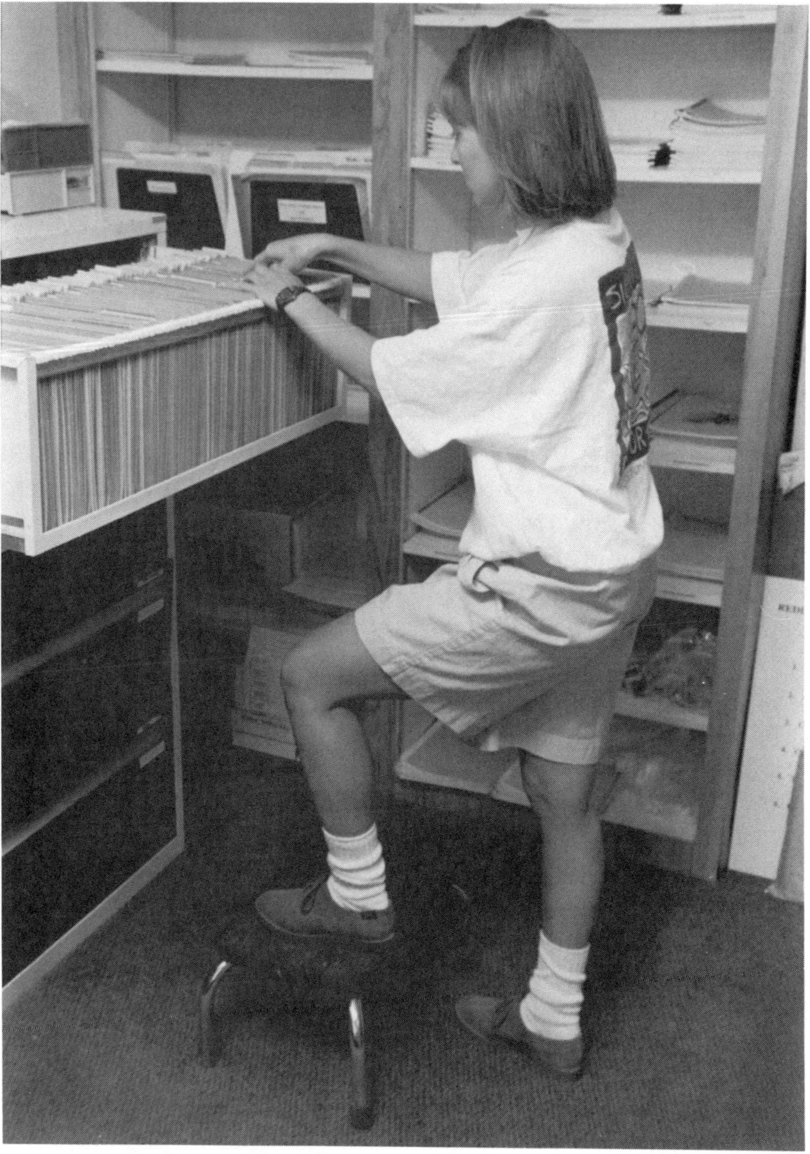

**Figure 5.2.** Propping one foot takes pressure off the spine.

the stomach. This may help with posture, especially in prevention of a stooped-over posture.

As your muscles become stronger with the regular exercise program (usually after a few weeks to a few months), your posture will improve without your thinking about it. Adding these simple measures to protect your back from unnecessary forces will give you even better results.

## What about Lifting?

Lifting does not have to be dangerous even when done regularly at work or at home. Know the facts about lifting so that you can protect your back from forces that increase the work it must do and, consequently, the chance of back pain and injury.

Did you know that very high forces are placed on the lower back when any of us lifts an object? Lifting an object weighing 86 pounds (39 kg), even with proper lifting techniques, can cause a force of over 700 pounds on the lower back discs! Heavier weights cause proportionally higher loads on the lower back. In light of these facts, it is surprising that injuries and back pain are not more common than they are.

We can't avoid many of our daily tasks, but we must become smart in the way we use our backs. The regular exercise program will continue to strengthen your back muscles. It makes sense that the stronger and more flexible the back muscles, the more they may be able to tolerate pressures. Proper lifting techniques can help minimize the forces we place on the back.

The following sections describe a few steps to keep in mind to help avoid back injuries when lifting. The National Institute for Occupational Safety and Health has given some of these recommendations for preventing injuries from lifting. We've added some other recommendations of our own.

### Lifting Technique

When you lift an object from the floor, you should be close to the object. Try to start with the center of the weight about seven or eight inches from your body. Try to hold the object close to your body, not at arm's length. Lifting with the arms held out puts higher amounts of stress on the back.

Try to lift with your legs and not your back. Using the strength of the legs helps to take some of the weight off the back muscles. These are easy but important ways to prevent back injuries when lifting.

The distance lifted should be no more than 12 to 13 inches for a weight above 86 pounds. If the weight is heavier, the distance lifted should be shorter. If the weight must be lifted higher, then assistance or a machine would be helpful. It is a good idea for work positions or loading platforms to be adaptable to the differing height and needs of the employees.

Try not to reach in order to lift objects higher than chest level. Lifting above chest level can cause much higher stress on the back muscles. If you must reach above your head to lift something, use a stool or ladder.

A weight of more than 86 pounds should be lifted carefully and no more frequently than every five minutes. This interval can't always be controlled. When you must lift more often, be sure to follow all other guidelines to prevent injury.

Never twist your back when lifting. Twisting puts much more force on the back. If you have to turn, pivot with your feet.

Always be sure of your footing. A sudden change in foot placement or a trip can cause a high amount of force on the back.

If the object you are lifting is too heavy, have someone else help you or use a mechanical lever or machine.

Always use both hands when lifting; more force is put on the back when you lift using only one hand. Sudden lifting, such as jerking the object upward, also causes a great increase in the back pressures. Try to make your lifts smooth and gradual to lower the work load on your back.

## Support Belts

Lower back (lumbar) support belts are used by weight lifters. The belts have been found by some researchers to help decrease the stress on the spine and back muscles when squatting and lifting. If you do heavy lifting in your job or if you must lift frequently, it may be helpful for you to use a lifting belt or other back support.

With continued lifting, the muscles of the back and abdomen may become tired and more likely to be injured, especially when lifting heavy loads. A lifting belt may give added support, helping to prevent injury after the muscles become more stressed and tired.

If your job demands only occasional lifting, a back support belt may not be necessary. If you feel more comfortable wearing a back support belt, it is acceptable to use. Remember that back supports can't replace proper lifting technique, and no support or lifting belt can substitute for a regular exercise program to strengthen the muscles of the back. Our basic exercise program should be continued twice daily for prevention.

## Other Factors

### On-the-Job Risk

Many experts have found that jobs that require frequent heavy lifting and similar routine duties may have a higher risk of back pain and injuries. If your job is repetitious or tedious and you have had a back injury, you should take special measures to strengthen your back muscles. Be sure to use proper lifting techniques, and take particular care that you do all you can to prevent back injuries. Your employer may be able to contribute to preventing back injuries by providing special safety equipment. Ideally, employers show concern for their workers by giving attention to individual needs in the workplace. Prevention education and evaluation of the job site can also guard against serious injuries.

Workers who feel dissatisfied with their jobs seem to be at higher risk for back pain. This situation may be difficult to deal with, but, if possible, try to eliminate those factors that are contributing to your dissatisfaction. This may be very difficult in some cases, without a job change.

## Stress

Back pain causes stress, and stress from other causes can make the back pain worse. In this vicious cycle of pain and stress, each makes the other worse. Pain caused by stress is not imagined; it is very real. Among the other medical problems that can be made worse by stress are the many types of arthritis.

Stress can disrupt other parts of your life, including the interpersonal relationships in your family and at work. The stress caused by back pain, with its loss of activity, loss of sleep, loss of income, and high expenses, can be devastating. These effects can be attacked and controlled, and steps can be taken to prevent and control stress later. Some easy ways to achieve these goals are discussed in Chapter Eight.

This chapter has described the factors that should be addressed to prevent future attacks of back pain. We find that those who are able to follow these guidelines are usually able to improve their control of attacks of acute back pain. For chronic back pain, these guidelines are even more important. They hope to prevent further injury and aggravation of present back pain.

CHAPTER SIX

# Get the Weight off Your Back

If you are too heavy, one of the most important steps you can take to eliminate your back pain is to lose weight. But let's face it—diets make us crazy. In any given year, 50 percent of all women in the United States and 25 percent of all men go on at least one diet. People diet for many reasons: to lose weight, to reduce cholesterol, to gain weight or muscle, to control diabetes, or, for those with back pain, to eliminate the constant, nagging pain caused by excess weight.

The diet business brings in tens of billions of dollars each year. People spend a lot of money trying to find the "perfect" diet. Informed people try to follow diets that are balanced, practical, and healthy. People looking for fast weight loss may adopt diets that are based on little research and have questionable results. Many people even lean toward diets that can be downright unhealthy and even dangerous.

Are we really achieving the weight loss we are spending all this money for? The answer is an emphatic *No!* Studies show that approximately 95 percent of people who go on weight-loss diets will gain all or some of the weight back. Many people will gain back more weight than they had lost. In fact, some studies have found that, after a period of five years, no one-time diet program was successful in keeping the weight off.

## How Diet Programs Can Set You Up for Failure

Most diet programs tell you what foods to eat, how much to eat, and when to eat it. You have very little flexibility; your diet is pretty much the same as the diet for the person sitting next to you at the program sessions, even though each of you has very different needs and desires. Another of our objections is that these programs emphasize losing weight. You may wonder, "Isn't that what I'm there for?" The answer is no. You should be there to learn how to *manage* your weight.

Most popular diet programs do help you lose weight, but we all know how to do that. The real problem is keeping the weight off. Even programs that have a life-style management or behavior modification component generally do not put the emphasis on this goal. Instead, losing weight is always the focus. It is not until the weight is lost that you begin to work on your eating habits. Unfortunately, this approach has had dismal success.

Those who have successfully lost weight focus on developing a permanent life-style change. They don't even worry about losing weight. By gradually changing their eating habits, they take small, easily attainable steps toward a healthier life-style. And guess what? They lose weight *and they keep it off.*

More importantly, they are able to maintain their new goal-weight because they have made a commitment to three simple goals:

1. They eat healthily.
2. They move their bodies more.
3. They do both for the rest of their lives.

Why aren't there "programs" that focus more on making life-style changes than on staying on any particular diet? The reason is economics. Results from the life-style approach come more slowly, and people who want to lose weight look for rapid results. Programs that promise and deliver rapid results are more salable. Dieters want to be able to eat anything they choose and still lose weight. If that option isn't part of a weight loss plan, they want someone to take away all responsibility for food choices from them and promise them quick results. That is the kind of attitude that keeps people fat.

Statistics show that from 25 percent to 64 percent of Americans are overweight. Studies indicate that men expect to lose three to four pounds per week, and women expect to lose two to three pounds per week. If they don't succeed with these weight-loss goals, many attendees will drop out of the program after the third visit. This has led to many programs' adopting a "quick start" regimen in which weight loss is more during the first few weeks. This is an enticement to start the program, but when the weight loss slows down, the honeymoon is over and discouragement sets in.

Once someone gets discouraged, feelings of failure are close behind. Only those people who are willing to work hard and make a lifetime commitment will have long-term success with weight loss.

Any "diet" will work if you have that commitment, provided that the diet includes choices from all the food groups. Diets that rely on liquid supplements or include only a limited number of foods can be the worst perpetrators of out-of-control eating. If you emphasize trying to lose weight rather than changing your life-style, you have not made a true weight loss commitment. Chances are you will join the 95 percent of dieters who fail at weight management.

In our clinic, we present our patients with many different approaches and allow them to choose the program that best suits their life-style. Among the options are: counting fat grams, counting calories, using food exchanges, eating low-fat and low-calorie frozen meals, or any other approach the patient may want to try. The only "bad diet" is *one that does not allow for real food in real situations and is not nutritionally well-balanced.* If a patient finds that the chosen approach does not work, we try other approaches until we find one that is right.

Studies indicate that people who devise their own plans for diet change are more likely to keep lost weight off. In a 1990 California study, 73 percent of the people who maintained their weight loss had devised their own plan of action, but only 39 percent of those who relapsed had done so. The self-choice approach works because people plan for the changes they are willing to make rather than be handed changes someone else has told them they should make.

## To Lose Weight, Quit Dieting

Our answer to the diet problem is to have our patients *quit dieting*. In our clinic, we assess each person's current diet and exercise habits. From that assessment, we determine what changes should be made, and the patients plan the changes that they are willing to make. Together, we establish a reasonable, healthy plan that requires gradual changes over time. In this way, each person "owns" his or her program and feels empowered to make changes toward a healthier life-style.

### Dieting Can Lead to Bingeing

Why do we advise people to quit dieting? Because, as we have already stated, dieting does not work. Among its other effects, dieting in the traditional sense can lead to bingeing. The frequency and size of each person's binges vary under different circumstances. Almost every dieter has, at some time, eaten a low-fat, low-calorie, nutritionally correct meal, then polished off the rest of the brownies later (usually when all alone).

Bingeing, even small bingeing, will make it difficult for you to lose weight because you will feel out of control and "bad." This will lead you to ask: "If I can control everything else in my life, why can't I control my eating?" The reason is that traditional diets forbid certain foods. What happens when you tell yourself you can't have a certain food? Take ice cream as an example. Suddenly, the off-diet ice cream becomes the food you desire most in the whole world. The urge to eat ice cream becomes uncontrollable, and you eventually give in and binge.

Dieting by forbidding certain foods is like holding your breath: you can only do it for so long. Eventually, you have to take a breath, and the first breath (a binge breath, if you will) is very deep. When this happens in dieting, you feel guilty and vow to avoid that troublesome food forever. This only sets you up for another binge.

## Dieting Can Make You Fatter

A third reason to avoid dieting is because it can make you fatter. Every time you lose ten pounds or more, especially if it's on a very low-calorie or quick-weight-loss diet, you lose muscle and fat. When you gain the weight back, it's usually just fat. This leaves you with more fat and less muscle each time you lose weight. This is like taking one step forward and two steps back.

When your body fat increases, your metabolism slows down, because, to maintain itself, fat requires little energy and fewer calories than does muscle. Fat is not a very active tissue; it stores itself until it is needed, which is only in a last-resort scenario. Not only do you gain more weight, but your calorie needs to maintain your weight become less with each diet. The next time you diet, it will take twice as long to lose the weight, and you will gain it back three times as fast.

## Dieting Can Be Hazardous to Your Overall Health and Your Heart

A final reason to avoid dieting is because it can be detrimental to your health. Results from the Framingham Heart Study, in Massachusetts, showed yo-yo dieters were twice as likely to suffer from heart disease as were overweight people who had stable weights.

When obesity is bad and dieting is bad, what are people to do? The challenging answer is: Quit dieting, eat healthily, exercise more, and make a commitment to permanent life-style changes.

## Use the New Food Guide Pyramid

How exactly does one eat healthily? The Food Guide Pyramid designed by the U.S. Departments of Agriculture and Health and Human Services is an excellent guideline for determining a healthy diet (see Figure 6.1). Most food choices should come from the lower part of the pyramid. These are the foods that contain complex carbohydrates—whole grain breads and cereals, pasta, rice and other grains, vegetables, and fruits.

Looking at the pyramid, you see starchy foods are at the bottom. Most of your calories should come from this group.

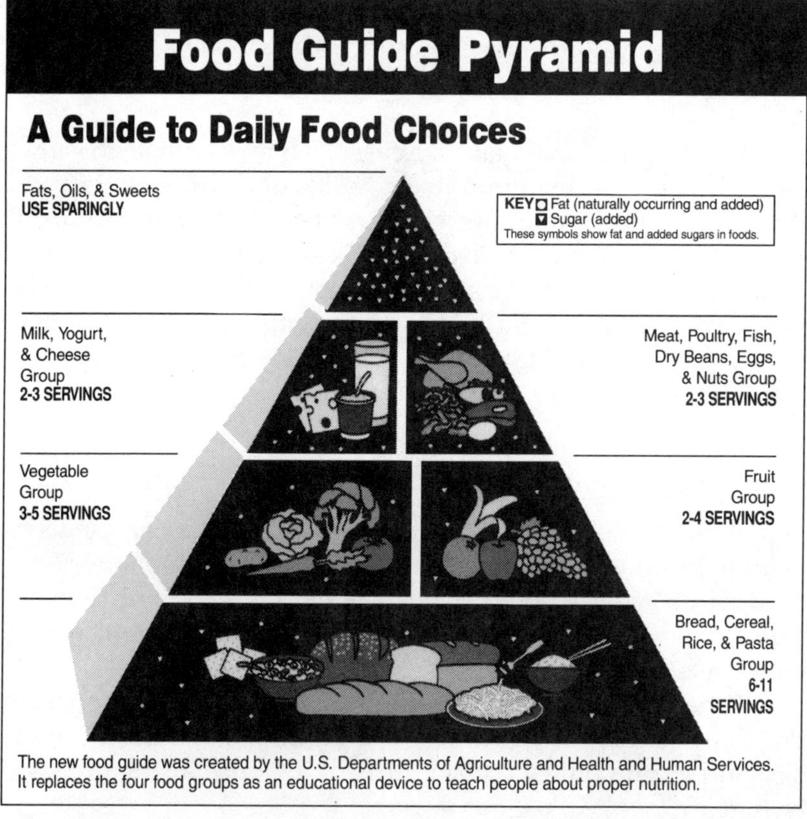


**Figure 6.1.** The Food Guide Pyramid: A guide to daily food choices.

Many people have difficulty accepting this, because they have grown up thinking starchy foods are "fattening."

Most traditional diets are low in carbohydrates (and high in protein), so there is widespread belief that carbohydrates are fattening. In fact, starches are low in fat, high in fiber, and packed with vitamins and minerals. More important in terms of weight loss, most people love them. As an extra plus, they are very satisfying and keep hunger away longer.

When you give up starches, you are setting yourself up for failure. Six to 11 servings per day are recommended. If you are trying to lose weight, eat the minimum number of servings recommended in each food group. Table 6.1 lists serving sizes of various starchy foods.

Fruits and vegetables are on the next level of the pyramid. "Five a Day for Good Health" is the slogan used to try to get people to eat more of these foods. Only 8 percent of the population know they should eat a minimum of two servings of fruits and three servings of vegetables each day. In fact, 34 percent of the population believe they should eat one or fewer servings of fruits and vegetables each day. The average American eats three-and-a-half servings each day.

Fruits and vegetables are packed with nutrients. They are also low-calorie and virtually fat-free. They even have the "crunch factor": crunchy foods are very satisfying to eat. Fruits and vegetables are definitely foods to be eaten in large quantities.

When we ask people about their intake of fruits and vegetables, their usual response is that they like them but they just don't think about them. It's time to think about them, even if you must make a note to yourself and tape it to your kitchen cabinets. (See Table 6.2 for the values in servings of fruits and vegetables.)

As you move up the pyramid, its area gets smaller, as do the number of servings recommended. This does not mean these foods are less important; we just don't need as much of them. In traditional diets, dairy foods, like starches, are among the first to go, because they are perceived to be fattening. Some people have a mistaken notion that they no longer need milk when they

**Table 6.1**
**Starchy Food Servings**

| Food | Serving Size | Calories | Fat (Grams) |
|---|---|---|---|
| Breads | 1 slice | 80 | 1 |
| Bagels | 1 small | 160 | 1.5 |
| English muffin | 1 small | 130 | 1 |
| Hamburger and hot dog rolls | 1 | 115 | 2 |
| Tortilla | 1 | 70 | 1 |
| Diet bread | 2 slices | 80 | 1 |
| Crackers | | | |
| Animal crackers | 8 | 80 | 1 |
| Arrowroot | 3 | 65 | 2 |
| Graham crackers | 2 squares | 60 | 1.5 |
| Saltines | 6 | 80 | 2 |
| Melba toast | 5 slices | 80 | 1 |
| Cereals, Grains, Pasta | | | |
| Cooked cereal | ½ cup | 80 | 0.5 |
| Instant/Flavored cooked cereal | 1 packet | 135 | 2 |
| Ready-to-eat dry cereal, unsweetened | 1 ounce | 110 | 1 |
| Granola | ¼ cup | 130 | 5 |
| Low-fat granola | ⅓ cup | 120 | 2 |
| Pasta | 1 cup | 160 | 0.5 |
| Popcorn, popped, no fat | 3 cups | 80 | 1 |
| Starchy Vegetables | | | |
| Corn | ½ cup | 80 | 1 |
| Peas | ½ cup | 60 | 0.5 |
| Potato, baked, with skin | 1 large | 220 | 0.5 |
| Winter squash | ½ cup | 60 | 0.5 |
| Sweet potatoes | ½ cup | 80 | 0 |

**Table 6.2**
**Fruit and Vegetable Servings**

| Food | Serving Size | Calories | Fat (Grams) |
|---|---|---|---|
| *Vegetables* | | | |
| All varieties other than starchy vegetables have approximately 25 calories and less than 1 gram fat per ½ cup cooked serving and 1 cup raw serving. | | | |
| *Fruits* | | | |
| Fresh fruit | 1 small piece | 60 | less than 1 |
| Canned fruit, no sugar added | ½ cup | 60 | less than 1 |
| Fruit juice | ½ cup | 60 | less than 1 |
| Dried fruit | ¼ cup | 60 | less than 1 |

reach adulthood. Dairy foods contribute important nutrients to the daily diet. They are especially important in building and maintaining strong, dense bones. The calcium found in dairy products is necessary in the prevention of osteoporosis, one of the causes of back pain (see page 20). Recent research also indicates the importance of calcium, potassium, and magnesium in the regulation of blood pressure. Dairy foods contain all three nutrients in abundance.

Two to three servings a day of dairy foods are recommended, or three to four if you have osteoporosis. A serving is one cup of milk or yogurt or one ounce of cheese. Use the low-fat or fat-free versions of these foods. (See Table 6.3 for a listing of the values of dairy foods.)

Some people have problems with the digestion of the milk carbohydrate, lactose, and may avoid all milk products for that reason. Symptoms of lactose intolerance include intestinal cramping, gas, and diarrhea. If you suffer from lactose intolerance and avoid milk products, be sure you get adequate calcium from other food sources or supplements. Special products available at most supermarkets and pharmacies can be added to your diet to counteract the lactose intolerance, making it possible for you to drink milk and enjoy milk products. Some milk products

**Table 6.3**
**Milk, Cheese, and Yogurt Servings**

| Food | Serving Size | Calories | Fat (Grams) |
|---|---|---|---|
| Skim milk | 1 cup | 90 | 1 |
| 1% fat milk | 1 cup | 100 | 2 |
| 2% fat milk | 1 cup | 120 | 5 |
| Whole milk | 1 cup | 150 | 8 |
| Goat milk | 1 cup | 170 | 10 |
| 1% fat buttermilk | 1 cup | 100 | 2 |
| Evaporated skim milk | ½ cup | 100 | 0.5 |
| Yogurt, plain | 1 cup | 130 | 0.5 |

are chemically treated to make them safe for people who have lactose intolerance. Be sure to read your dairy product labels to learn which ones are low-fat, low-calorie, and treated for lactose intolerance.

Protein foods are a food group that Americans eat in larger amounts than the body needs. (Possible exceptions are dried beans, peas, and lentils.) Protein is needed to build and maintain body tissues, and many people think if a little is good for building muscle, then a lot must build even more muscle. That is not the case.

Body builders need a slightly higher amount than the average person, but, with most Americans eating double or triple the needed amount of protein, that is hardly an issue. If you eat more protein than you need, the excess will be burned as energy, if needed, or stored, if not needed immediately. Four to six ounces, or the equivalent, per day are all you need for good health. Protein foods contain fat, so it is a good idea to limit these foods to their recommended levels. (See Table 6.4 for a listing of the values of meats and meat substitutes, the leading protein foods consumed in America.)

At the top of the pyramid, in the smallest section, are fats, oils, and sweets. The advice is "Use sparingly," but what does that mean? If you are trying to lower your cholesterol but are not worried about your weight, you should have no more than

**Table 6.4**
**Meats and Meat Substitutes**

| Food | Serving Size | Calories | Fat (Grams) |
|---|---|---|---|
| Low-fat meats | 3 ounces, cooked | 165 | 9 |
| Medium-fat meats | 3 ounces, cooked | 225 | 15 |
| High-fat meats | 3 ounces, cooked | 300 | 24 |

25 grams added fat in your daily diet. Alcohol, which is metabolized in a manner similar to fat, should be limited as well.

If you are trying to lose weight, you should eat no more than 15 grams of added fat. This fat level does not include fat that occurs naturally in foods such as lean meat, fish, poultry, low-fat cheese, and other low-fat dairy products, but it does include fat that you or the food manufacturers add to your food.

Butter, margarine, cooking oil, salad dressing, mayonnaise, and fats cloaked in chemical disguises are added to snack foods, desserts, and other packaged foods.

The recommended amounts are: no more than one small serving per day for women or two small servings per day for men. (See Table 6.5 for a listing of the values of fat servings.)

Many people believe that to stay on their diet and to eat healthily, they must not eat cookies, candies, or other desserts.

**Table 6.5**
**Fats Servings**

| Food | Serving Size | Calories | Fat (Grams) |
|---|---|---|---|
| Margarine, mayonnaise, oil, butter | 1 teaspoon | 45 | 5 |
| Diet margarine and mayonnaise | 1 Tablespoon | 45 | 5 |
| Salad dressing | 1 Tablespoon | 60 | 5 |
| Diet salad dressing | 2 Tablespoons | 60 | 5 |
| Sour cream | 2 Tablespoons | 50 | 5 |
| Light sour cream | 2 Tablespoons | 35 | 2 |
| Cream cheese | 1 Tablespoon | 50 | 5 |
| Light cream cheese | 1 Tablespoon | 30 | 3 |

There are no good foods and no forbidden foods—only foods you should eat more of and foods you should eat less of. One small dessert one to three times per week will not make you obese nor will it sabotage your diet efforts.

One equation says it all for long-lasting weight reduction:

Reduce fat = Reduce weight

Reducing fat in the diet is an effective strategy for losing weight because a lot of calories can be eliminated without having to reduce the volume of food consumed. With nine calories per gram of fat and only four calories per gram of protein or carbohydrate, fat is the most concentrated source of calories in most people's diet. Alcohol, which has seven calories per gram, is in second place.

Excess fat has been linked to heart disease, some cancers, and obesity. Women especially seem to benefit from reducing fat intake to lose weight.

## What about Supplements?

Can you get the nutrients you need from sources other than food? You can take food supplements, and many people do, but supplements are not a substitute for a well-balanced diet. Supplements contain only those nutrients we know are essential and have an established recommended daily allowance or safe and effective level. There is still much we don't know about the nutrients our bodies need.

Food provides nutrients we know about, as well as those we don't know about. Our bodies use nutrients more efficiently if they are provided in small amounts throughout the day, rather than in a single dose.

Supplements that provide 100 percent of the recommended daily allowances (RDAs) are safe and may be helpful for certain populations, such as the elderly or the very young, if taken as supplements. It is still essential to eat a healthy, balanced diet. Be careful of "megadoses" of specific vitamins or minerals.

They can be dangerous and may interfere with the work of other nutrients.

### Your Plan of Action

Once you have determined your diet and life-style goals, you need a plan of action—a set of strategies you can use to help you achieve your goals. Table 6.6 contains tried-and-true strategies to help you in almost any situation. Look over the list and highlight the solutions you are willing to try. In your mind, practice using them in different situations. The more you practice them ahead of time, the easier it will be to use them in real crises.

## Exercise Regularly for Weight Loss and a Healthy Back

Exercise is an essential component in any weight management program. Without exercise, weight management for life is nearly impossible to achieve. "But I hate to exercise," you may say. "I don't like to sweat." Comments like these are very common. Overweight people tend to be much less active than their thin counterparts. You do not need to join a gym or buy expensive workout equipment or clothing. Just move more often and more quickly than you normally do. Walk whenever and wherever you can. Make exercise as much a part of your day as brushing your teeth.

Scheduling a time for exercise helps. If you have a dedicated time and place, you will be more likely to follow through. Look at your daily routine and pinpoint blocks of time suitable for exercise. TV time is good, as is the 15 minutes you stay in bed after your alarm goes off. Consider splitting the exercise time into three ten-minute sessions. It's a lot easier to find ten minutes than a half-hour.

Try to do your regular activities at a higher level of intensity. Put more effort into your housework. Turn on some lively music; it will help you move faster. You'll also get more work done!

**Table 6.6**
**Solutions to Diet Pitfalls**

1. Don't get fatigued; keep regular hours.
2. Never allow yourself to get too hungry; do not skip meals.
3. Keep low-calorie, low-fat foods on hand and within easy reach.
4. Take a snack pack to work to ease temptation at break time, or eat on the way home so you don't arrive starving.
5. If you are tempted to buy a high-calorie food at the supermarket, carry home a five-pound bag of sugar instead.
6. Always start your meal with a low-calorie, high-volume food such as a clear soup, or fruit, or a vegetable salad.
7. Never go to a party hungry; be like Scarlett O'Hara and eat something first.
8. Never sit near the snack table at a party.
9. Offer to bring a low-fat appetizer to a party and be your own best customer.
10. Decide which treats are really important to you, then plan for the times you will allow yourself to eat them.
11. Plan gatherings around activities other than food, such as board games or yard games.
12. Measure foods, especially added-fat and protein foods, for appropriate portion sizes.
13. Use a smaller plate.
14. Put on your plate the amount you usually would eat, then remove half and store it for another meal.
15. Share your serving with another person.
16. Never eat alone.
17. Preplan and schedule meals and snacks so you are never so hungry that you lose control.
18. Take a nap when you crave a snack.
19. Preplan an enjoyable activity for times when you have difficulty controlling your eating.
20. Drink a glass of water before eating anything.
21. Keep low-calorie foods on hand and visible; hide or throw out high-calorie foods.
22. Eat only when you are truly hungry.
23. Keep a food diary.
24. Ask yourself if you really want the food.
25. Set a timer for 20 minutes any time you get the urge to eat. In that time, ask yourself: Do I really want to eat? What do I want to eat? How much shall I take? In this way, even if you decide to eat

**Table 6.6** *(Continued)*

something, you have given yourself a chance to manage your eating instead of letting it control you.

26. Eat only at scheduled times.
27. Keep foods on hand that require preparation—no convenience foods.
28. Stop eating when you are full.
29. Take at least 20 minutes for each meal; set a timer if you need to.
30. Chew your food thoroughly.
31. Eat foods high in fiber; they require more chewing and they fill your stomach.
32. Put your utensils down between bites; don't pick them up until you have swallowed the previous bite.
33. Cut your food in smaller pieces.
34. Fill your plate at the stove; do not keep extra food on the table.
35. Put leftovers in the refrigerator immediately after serving.
36. Leave the table immediately after finishing a meal: Do not sit in front of the TV; plan an activity to keep you busy.
37. Buy a calorie book.
38. Find a satisfying low-calorie food to substitute for high-calorie foods.
39. Read labels for fat, chemicals, and calorie content; pay attention to serving sizes.
40. Avoid purchasing tempting foods too often; plan for the times when you will purchase them.
41. Use relaxation, visualization, and assertiveness techniques to help practice for success in handling difficult situations.
42. Make strong, positive statements about yourself and your goals.
43. Keep a journal of events that trigger your eating. Supply a plan of action to avoid each trigger.
44. Separate stress and other emotional issues from eating.
45. Find nonfood ways to reward yourself.
46. Ask people not to give you food as gifts.
47. Learn to say "no" gracefully and assertively, with no reference to your diet; you do not have to justify your actions. Practice saying "no" in front of the mirror.
48. Arrange your household activities so you do not have to go into the kitchen very often.
49. Limit your eating to a few designated eating areas that are free from other distractions.
50. Exercise during TV food and beverage commercials, or leave the room (but avoid the kitchen).

**Table 6.6** *(Continued)*

51. Avoid routes that take you past places that sell foods that tempt you.
52. Cook with a flavored toothpick in your mouth or chew gum.
53. Brush your teeth when you get the urge to eat at an inappropriate time.
54. Decide what you will eat before you enter a restaurant.
55. Do not engage in other activities, such as reading, driving, watching TV, and so on, while you are eating.
56. Take your diet one day at a time; make a fresh resolution each day to eat healthily.
57. Set objective, action-oriented goals, not just weight-loss goals.
58. Take up a hobby, listen to music, dance.
59. Take a class, preferably one that is in session during your most difficult time of the day.
60. Do some volunteer work.
61. Diet with a friend.
62. Always eat off a dish, not out of a package.
63. Find or create a "fat" picture or cartoon of yourself and a picture or cartoon of how you want to look. Display it where you will see it every day.
64. Always eat sitting down.
65. Fill an activities jar with slips of paper on which you've written your chores, errands, current dress or shirt size, household maintenance jobs, letters you should answer, pleasant future activities, favorite movie titles, CDs you want, music group names, hobbies, and so on. Reach into this jar for distraction instead of reaching for food.
66. Make a list of ten reasons why you want to reach your goal; keep it handy and look at it to reinforce your commitment to weight management.
67. Look at your planned activities for the week and preplan how you will handle each different eating situation.
68. Do not keep eating until you are "stuffed."
69. Limit your intake of coffee, tea, alcohol, and diet beverages; they may stimulate the desire to eat.
70. Add more high-fiber, low-fat bulk to your meals.
71. Exercise regularly.
72. Do not shop for food before meals or when you are hungry or tired.
73. Eat a dill pickle.

Many people walk in malls. This location is especially beneficial for people who may be afraid to walk far in their neighborhoods. Many malls have walking programs set up with trails and distance markers.

Another way you can increase your exercise is to use stairs instead of an elevator. Start off one floor below your intended floor. As you feel more comfortable, gradually increase the number of flights you walk. You're on the first or second floor? No problem! Walk up a few extra flights, then walk down to the floor you need to be on. It is also helpful to combine exercise with passive activities. Read your mail while riding your stationary bike; stretch while you watch TV.

Remember, exercise is an essential component of your weight management strategy. We have discussed (1) changing your eating habits, (2) exercising, and (3) staying with those two rules for the rest of your life. We guarantee that if you adopt those three recommendations, you *will* manage your weight for life. We also guarantee that if you leave out one of them, your chances of lifetime management are very slim.

CHAPTER SEVEN

# Nonstandard Treatments

As long as there is back pain, there will be nonstandard treatments. Nonstandard treatments often offer quick relief or cure, are usually easy to do, and, most importantly, usually have not been tested as required by the U.S. Food and Drug Administration (FDA) for new treatments.

Nonstandard treatments are often passed along through the years by word of mouth. Or, they may be treatments proposed as new "miracle cures." The latest nonstandard treatments are often reported in the grocery store tabloids with sensational headlines such as "Scientist Finds New Cure for Back Pain" or "Once-a-Day Pill Cures Aching Back." They are often touted as good treatments that have been covered up or overlooked by doctors or other groups. Don't believe everything you read.

Some people try these treatments because they are frustrated over their constant back pain. It is hard to turn down what seems like a quick and easy solution. You can try these remedies if they are harmless and will not delay proper diagnosis and treatment. You may feel better knowing that you have not missed an easy answer to your pain.

Some nonstandard treatments are not harmful or expensive, and they can be easily added to a basic treatment program for back pain. Like chicken soup, they won't hurt and might help. But remember to keep up the basic treatment program as well.

Following are the questions you should ask before using any nonstandard treatment for back pain:

- How old is the treatment, what tests have been done, and what might be the side effects?
- What does the treatment cost?
- How long should it take to feel relief?

From the answers, you can judge whether the treatment will work for you.

There are countless nonstandard treatments for chronic back pain. Let's look at some of those that are most common.

Many treatments for chronic back pain are actually treatments for arthritis in the lower back. There are over 100 different types of arthritis, and treatment is not the same for every type. Most nonstandard treatments are probably intended to treat osteoarthritis, the wear-and-tear arthritis.

## Dietary Treatments

Many diet remedies for back pain are traceable to the fact that some patients feel better or worse when they eat certain foods and avoid others. Some patients feel their arthritis and back pain worsen when they eat tomato products, citrus fruits, and red meat, among other foods. Some people claim they feel better when they decrease their intake of proteins, carbohydrates, or total calories. In treatment for arthritis causing chronic back pain, folk medicine diets exclude white flour and all sweets except honey. Diets such as these are generally healthy and are certainly not harmful.

The truth is that there are no proven ways to affect osteoarthritis in the back by changes in diet. We suggest that if your arthritis and back pain improve when you eat or omit certain foods, then a trial of a few months may be worthwhile. If you find relief in your case, you can continue the plan.

## Omega-3

One specific diet item that has benefited some patients with pain from arthritis is the addition of Omega-3 fatty acids, which are found in fish oil from herring and certain other fish. Some people find that pain and stiffness may improve after a few months of taking supplement capsules of EPA (eicosapentaenoic acid) or eating several servings of herring weekly. No serious side effects are known when Omega-3 is taken in moderate amounts.

## Vitamin Supplements

Various vitamins and minerals have also been suggested as effective for treatment of arthritis in the back and chronic back pain. No specific evidence favors any single vitamin or mineral supplement. If you do take vitamins or minerals to relieve arthritis in the back, take only the recommended daily allowance (RDA) as suggested by the American Dietetics Association. Some vitamins and minerals can be very harmful if ingested in large amounts. If in doubt, ask your physician or nutritionist.

## Creams, Lotions, and Liniments

Creams, lotions, and liniments are widely advertised for the relief of back pain and other conditions. Research does not show that there is a definite advantage to these treatments, but they are not harmful when used properly, and they can be continued if you feel improvement in back pain. Many types of creams, lotions, and rubs are available over-the-counter.

## DMSO (Dimethyl Sulfoxide)

DMSO (dimethyl sulfoxide) is a liquid available for application to the skin. It has been used for treatment of injuries to muscles and tendons, but is dangerous if taken internally. DMSO is absorbed through the skin and causes a garlic-breath odor. It is not recommended; after some popularity, its use has declined over the past few years. Some patients feel that it gives temporary relief of pain when it is applied. If you use DMSO, you should be careful to use gloves so none is absorbed through the skin of the hands.

## Herbal Remedies

Herbal remedies have been used for generations and can be prepared in tea or soup, or taken in other forms. Certain remedies such as alfalfa are popular in some areas of this country. Most are not harmful, but none has been shown to have a specific benefit.

## Spas

The use of spas is one of the oldest treatments for arthritis and back pain sufferers. The Romans built elaborate baths to provide warm pools for treatment. The moist heat provided relief just as it does in today's treatments. Many age-old spas are still active and offer exercise and relaxation for their users. Modern spas, not necessarily built at natural springs, feature whirlpools, massage schedules, physical therapy, state-of-the-art exercise equipment, and support groups.

## Prayer and Meditation

Prayer has been used by arthritis sufferers with chronic back pain. In some surveys, roughly 40 percent of the respondents used prayer for help with pain. In one survey, over half of the respondents rated prayer as very helpful.

Many more nonstandard treatments are available, and new ones are created and reborn each year. If you have questions, ask your doctor's advice about your chances for benefit and the possible side effects of new or unusual treatments. There's nothing wrong with benefiting as early as possible from successful new developments, but you must protect yourself from adverse side effects of unproven remedies.

CHAPTER EIGHT

# Relieve Stress to Help End Your Back Pain

Back pain causes more than suffering within your body: It can also make your emotional state very fragile. Back pain can create stress in many ways, especially when the pain is unceasing and lasts for months. To the patient with back pain, the suffering seems never-ending:

- It prevents sleep at night, and the sleeplessness causes fatigue and irritability.
- It can make concentration and activity at work more difficult.
- If work must be stopped because of the back pain, then the loss of income, the loss of self-respect, the increased costs of care, and related problems add a high degree of stress.

How do high levels of stress cause more "wear and tear" on the body? The inactivity caused by the pain makes the muscles weaken. More tiredness, more fatigue, more unhappiness, and more stress result. The effect of back pain on a person's well-being becomes a vicious cycle of pain, fatigue, stress, then more pain, tiredness, unhappiness, and on.

Back pain stress can aggravate or even create other medical problems. If you have chronic back pain, stress can lead to more frequent and intense pain and can make it harder to handle other problems created by this suffering.

## The Stress of Back Pain

People with chronic back pain are faced with special demands and pressures because their illness may require changes in life-style or daily habits. Pain is the most common symptom experienced by back pain patients. The task of coping with daily pain often leads to stress that can actually make the pain more frequent and intense. When you are in pain, the body has a natural tendency to tighten up—muscles can become tense and rigid, causing additional strain and pressure on areas that were already painful. The cycle begins again with more pain.

Chronic back pain, along with other problems such as loss of independence, work adjustment difficulties, and worry about the future can combine to cause depression and other emotional reactions that further limit your ability to deal effectively with daily living. Depression is not a weakness—it is a common response to chronic stress in which people come to feel helpless.

## Signs and Symptoms of Stress

Stress is the word used to describe the many demands and pressures that all people experience to some degree each day. These demands may be physical or emotional in nature, and they require us to change or adapt in some fashion. For example, being stuck in slow-moving traffic requires that we change our expectations about arriving at our destination at an expected time. Similarly, the stress of going through a critical job interview requires that we do our best to maintain a relaxed, self-assured, and confident approach and make a good impression.

Stress can show itself through a wide variety of physical changes and emotional responses. Stress symptoms vary greatly from one person to the next. Perhaps the most universal sign of stress is a feeling of being pressured or overwhelmed. Some other signs and symptoms of stress are:

- Chronic fatigue;
- Loss of interest or enjoyment;
- Difficulty in concentration;
- Muscle tension;
- Impatience;
- Irritability or "easy anger";
- Difficulty sleeping;
- Change in appetite;
- Nervousness, edginess;
- Withdrawal;
- Trembling, sweaty hands.

If you recognize many or most of the stress characteristics in yourself, chances are good that your level of stress is excessive.

Maria, a 34-year-old woman, came to our clinic with chronic back pain and a dissolving marriage. Not only did her back hurt 24 hours a day, her personality had also changed greatly. "I've lost 12 pounds, and I was underweight to begin with," she said. "I can't sleep at night, and I feel so sensitive all day, like I could cry at the least little disruption. My husband won't speak to me because he is afraid I'll snap at him. I think our marriage is over, and it's my fault."

Maria's symptoms of weight loss, insomnia, and irritability were the result of the stress of back pain on her body. They were very real symptoms; she did not imagine them. When Maria was able to find relief from her chronic pain and begin the basic treatment plan as outlined in Chapter 3, she could begin to work on dealing with her stress. Maria saw a therapist who specializes in patients with chronic pain, and she began to understand her emotional state. Her husband joined her for family counseling, and now they are working at saving their marriage.

We saw another patient at the clinic who had lost his job because of the stress of his back pain. "No one knows how much pain I was in each day," Raymond, age 41, said. "I was the manager of a small appliances store and had to deal with people problems each day. All I heard was complaints and demands from the customers. I couldn't take it anymore. It was like the more demanding my customers became, the more edgy and irritable I became. They [the owners] told me to take a leave of absence until I could get some self-control. What am I going to do?"

After some intense therapy and instruction in how to handle his new stress level, Raymond finally returned to work recently. He is now beginning to control his back pain with a basic treatment plan instead of allowing his back pain to control him.

Learning to identify the ways in which your body and mind show stress is the first step in "managing the self" and reducing both your external demands and pressures and those you place on yourself.

With chronic back pain, you experience stressors across all aspects of your life, including:

- Physical stressors (the pain);
- Social stressors (loss of friends and activities);
- Work stressors (loss of job or difficulty working);
- Family stressors (feeling of dependency of others).

You have every right to be stressed, but you can do something about it.

## Coping Strategies for Decreasing Stress

Coping strategies *do* work! Take advantage of the available information and classes in your community as you find ways to reduce and *control* your stress level. Here are some suggestions:

1. Enroll in a stress management class or seminar (inquire at your local community mental health center).
2. Consult your doctor if you are experiencing physical symptoms of stress, such as high blood pressure, headaches, or anxiety attacks.

3. Get a referral for an individual counselor who might be helpful in teaching you to relax and manage your specific stress.
4. Consider special techniques, such as biofeedback, to provide you with tools to lower body tension or raise temperature levels.
5. Invest in stress management books and relaxation tapes that are available at local bookstores and music shops. Your library may have some of them for you to evaluate before you buy.
6. Examine your life carefully. Make a comprehensive list of all the things that stress you out. Eliminate or avoid stress sources that are not absolutely necessary. Try to modify the others.

## Dealing with Pain-Related Stress

People with chronic back pain typically deal with pain on a daily basis. The reason for their pain is genuine—there is something wrong in the body. The last thing you want to hear is, "I think it might be a good idea for you to speak with someone about your stress." You might immediately conclude that the "someone" is a psychiatrist, psychologist, or counselor of some type—more commonly known as a "shrink." You may be offended by the implication that the pain is "in your head." You may even become suspicious that this would-be adviser does not believe that you are really feeling the degree of pain in the back you describe.

If this has already happened to you or if it happens in the future, take a minute to explore your thoughts so that you can approach this subject in a rational manner. Let's examine some of the thoughts you may have.

### "No One Believes I Am in Pain"

"He thinks I'm making up my back pain." A middle-aged mother of three told us about her husband recently. "I guess

I'm so active raising the children, people would assume that I'm not in pain. But, honestly, I hurt all the time—when I get up, all day, when I go to bed at night."

It is very unlikely that your spouse, physician, friend, or anyone else who has recommended that you receive help believes you are not in pain. If you immediately become defensive and imagine the worst, this throws up roadblocks to any help you could receive by considering the impact of your emotional state on your pain. Back pain is real—no one should dispute that fact. Do not allow yourself to avoid the possibility of lessening the pain by assuming that others disbelieve or underrate your pain.

## "No One Understands Me"

"She doesn't understand what it is like to be in pain like this," another patient said. "My wife gets dressed each day and goes to work while I sit in my chair all day, barely able to move. I want to work, believe me. I feel so alone."

Those who are suggesting that you see a counselor may not have experienced the day-to-day debilitating pain that you constantly endure. However, lack of personal experience does not mean that their suggestions are not valid. Experienced professionals have formed a base of knowledge over the years, and they have seen the positive results of gaining control over emotions. They do not have to feel exactly as you do to make a valid recommendation for your welfare.

## "They Think I'm Not Trying"

"He thinks I could do more if I tried." Many patients we see tell us how they assume that friends and family members feel they are not trying to live with their pain. You *know* you have tried, and you are likely to be turned off by any implication that you have not put forth enough effort. Often, this is an interpretation that you have placed on the situation. You are trying, but you may not have tried or worked at your emotions from the standpoint that you can be in control. By changing your thinking, you can change your perception of the pain.

## The Role of Psychology in Chronic Back Pain

All comprehensive inpatient and outpatient chronic back pain programs include a psychological or behavioral component. It is widely accepted that emotional status can affect both the perception of pain and the ability to develop appropriate coping strategies.

All people with pain have stress. The stress makes it difficult for them to handle everyday issues, much less crisis situations that may arise. One patient who was in severe pain when we saw her admitted, "I realize that I'm moody, irritable, and even difficult to get along with. I tell my friends that this is the new me." Another patient with chronic back pain described her personality as "Dr. Jekyll and Mr. Hyde."

"I even warn my friends when I start to feel irritable or stressed out," she said laughing. "I tell them to stay away from me because I'm having a bad day."

The role of psychological counseling in a pain management program is to help the individual develop appropriate and workable coping strategies to deal with all of these issues. Psychological intervention is an accepted component for everyone—not just people who have "psychological problems."

Psychological intervention can provide you with coping methods that you can use either within or outside other treatment programs. In most cases, it is important that the therapist performing these services be trained in the area of pain management. Some of these options are described in the following sections.

### Individual Counseling

This is a one-on-one session with a therapist in which individual problem areas are addressed. The session may include specific help with alleviating depression, anxiety, or stress, along with several other problem areas addressed more specifically later in this chapter.

## Family Counseling

Back pain extends beyond the patient and can affect the entire family. It is often a good idea for family members to be involved in understanding your limitations and their possible impact on your family's life-style. Family members can have the best of intentions, but, without specific guidance, they sometimes make things worse. Family meetings are a forum for helping everyone deal with the stress of your chronic back pain and disability.

John and Amee told of benefiting greatly from family counseling. "When John injured his back at work and began to have chronic back pain, our family life was almost destroyed," Amee told us. "His anger and resentment of his condition reflected in the children's behavior at school and at home. I was torn apart trying to make a living for all of us while keeping up the housework, taking care of the kids, and being compassionate toward John. We almost didn't make it."

After several months of family counseling, John and Amee were able to work out their new situation and balance the stress level in their relationship. The good news is that John reported at his last visit that "Everything is better than before."

## Group Counseling

There is no one who can better understand your pain than another person with chronic back pain. Group sessions allow for the sharing of feelings and the development of effective coping strategies. Sandra, a 50-year-old woman, found great support in group counseling. "I feel emotionally healthy now," she said. "My group session meets every Monday night and allows me the opportunity to share my success and optimism with others. Of course, I also tell them about my bad days too! Somehow, my bad days always seem brighter after telling the persons in my group—they've had days like this as well."

This give-and-take at group meetings is often the most productive way to revamp your thought processes.

## Biofeedback

Relaxation is an accepted form of managing stress. Many chronic back pain programs teach patients to relax in order to reduce their pain levels. This can be accomplished with progressive relaxation or with the use of a medical technique called biofeedback.

With biofeedback, you are connected to a machine that informs you and your therapist when you are physically relaxing your body. The tension in your muscles, the amount of sweat produced, or the measurement of finger temperature are all indicators. Any one or all of these readings can let the trained biofeedback therapist know whether you are learning to relax.

The skill of relaxing can then be used outside the therapist's office when you encounter the day-to-day stresses of life. For practice of relaxation techniques, some therapists recommend relaxation tapes that can be listened to at home.

## Emotional and/or Behavioral Areas to Address in Pain Management

People with chronic back pain tend to have similar problems even though the structures of families are different and individual tolerances for pain runs from high to low endurance.

Many people with back pain feel frustrated at having become less agile. Tasks that were once easy—carrying out the garbage or bringing in bags of groceries—are now impossible. At times, their efforts to get up from a low or soft chair may be embarrassing. Even sexual activity can be difficult or painful. One young man told us that he was going to ask his wife for a divorce because of sexual problems after he injured his back in a sports accident. "I felt useless," he said. "I was in so much pain and didn't know how to solve it."

Fear becomes a great issue as people question what will happen in the future. Patients ask, "Will I have to give up many activities that I now enjoy" or "What will my family do?"

It is not fun to be in pain. At their most frustrated moments, some of our patients have even said that "a life with pain is no life at all." Your problems are real and are often devastating to your outlook on life and your daily activities. By going through some of these negative areas, you can learn effective coping techniques that lead to a positive winning attitude.

Read each of the following topical sections with an open mind, and explore ways in which you can make an impact in your life. There are alternatives to relying only on the medical treatment discussed elsewhere in this book, especially when many of the other avenues have not given complete relief. Not every problem area may apply to your own situation. We do, however, recommend that you read and think carefully about each emotion discussed. It may be something that you will have to face in the future, or it may help you help others.

## Anger and Irritability

You may be asking yourself, "Why me? Why should I have a life of misery with back pain? Why am I being punished or what have I done to deserve this?" Most people feel some degree of anger at the fact that they have to suffer with chronic back pain. Some use the anger in a positive manner, some ignore the anger, and some let these angry feelings consume their whole being. You should try to better understand your feelings of anger. Replace the energy you spend being angry with positive actions to make your life pleasurable.

## Understanding Anger

There are various forms of anger that people under stress from back pain may experience:

- *Upfront anger* is expressed directly toward the person or situation at which you are really angry. This type of anger, if not belabored or violent, is most acceptable.
- *Displaced anger* originates from strong feelings toward one person or event, but is directed toward another person or event. For example, your doctor may have suggested that you see a counselor to help you learn to relax. This

suggestion that the pain "might be in your head" makes you furious. Instead of screaming at the doctor, you scream at your spouse, expressing displaced anger.

- *Inward anger* is not expressed, either verbally or nonverbally. Instead of speaking about your anger, you let it boil up inside and eat away at your whole being.

You have a right to be angry, but you do not have a right to devastate yourself and others while expressing this anger. By holding on to angry feelings, you prevent yourself from moving forward to a more positive outlook.

## Coping Strategies for Anger and Irritability

If you are experiencing anger and irritability as your stress level increases, let the following suggestions help you work through this experience and move forward to a more relaxed frame of mind:

1. Accept the fact that anger is a human emotion that you are entitled to feel at times.
2. If anger is consuming your entire day, come to grips with the fact that you need to explore some avenues for behavior change. This may involve seeing a professional, talking out your reaction with a friend, or joining with others in the same situation to talk through your feelings.
3. Remember that constantly being angry is detrimental to your overall health.
4. When anger gets out of control, apologize to those you may have hurt.
5. Whenever possible, do not let yourself get into situations that you know will be unpleasant.
6. Ask your physician for a referral to a professional who can assist you in relaxing and reducing the tension that occurs from anger.

## Loss of Independence

Chronic back pain often leads to a loss of independence in your life. The degree of this loss varies with the frequency of pain, the intensity of pain, and your personality. We all have different tolerance levels and methods of handling our problems.

If you have always relied on other people, the entrance of chronic back pain into your life has probably increased your level of dependence. You may even have found this very comfortable. But your family may be feeling overwhelmed by your needs.

On the other hand, you may have prided yourself on never having to rely on others. If so, having to give up some of this self-sufficiency has probably destroyed your self-image. You may even find yourself going without some necessities just because you will not ask someone else to help.

## Coping Strategies for Loss of Independence

If you are experiencing a loss of independence, taking control of your abilities—even with chronic back pain—can help you regain some independence and self-esteem. Try these strategies:

1. Think about the activities you have stopped. Determine which ones are physically impossible, and which ones you are avoiding because of pain.
2. If you are doing everything you are physically capable of doing, don't feel guilty about asking for assistance with the things you absolutely cannot do.
3. Each week, try to do something new that you had been asking others to do for you.
4. If you have the financial means, hire the services you need instead of relying on family members. Your family may be very willing to help, but, over time, this dependency can lead them—and you—to feel some resentment.
5. Never let your family think you equate their love with the amount of help they give.
6. Never use guilt to make your family feel that they are not doing enough to help you.
7. Remember that the more you can do for yourself, the better you will feel about yourself.

## Loss of Control

Losing some independence isn't the only way you may feel loss of control over your life. You may now find that your activities no longer depend to the same extent on your intelligence, financial ability, perseverance, or desire. This realization cannot be easily understood by those who have not experienced the debilitating effect of chronic back pain.

## Coping Strategies for Loss of Control

Learning how to cope with chronic back pain and the loss of control you might feel does not have to be overwhelming. Look at the following suggestions and see how you can incorporate them into your daily life:

1. Determine which things you can control and make positive steps toward controlling them, rather than dwelling on your lack of control in other areas.
2. Make a list of things you want to change, then divide them into these two categories:

   THOSE THINGS I CAN CONTROL
   THOSE THINGS I CANNOT CONTROL

   With the help of a therapist, family members, or friends, begin to work on the things you can control.
3. If you find yourself becoming extremely agitated or stressed over a situation that is beyond your control, try to refocus your thoughts. If this does not work, ask for help from a professional.
4. Never consider yourself weak if you think you need help dealing with the loss of control. Those who refuse to ask for help are the weak ones. Knowing when to ask for help is, in fact, helping yourself.
5. Start working each week on a new action that will help you gain control. If you have trouble deciding what these actions should be, ask a counselor or a trusted friend to help you prioritize your list of actions that are possibly within your control. You might start by taking control of

your personal needs—bathing and dressing each day. Once you are able to fully take care of these needs, begin to take control of your home environment—cook one meal a day, clean your bedroom, or fold towels. Continue taking on new actions until you are able to accomplish most of your living needs without increased pain and discomfort.

6. Throw your pessimistic attitude away. You can gain better control, but you must work at it.

## Denial

The ultimate goal you can hope to achieve with chronic back pain is to reach the point where you can live with the condition and are ready to make modifications to handle it within your life. The flip side of this acceptance is *denial.* Denial works at complete odds with any type of rehabilitation effort. If you are not willing to admit that nonmedical issues such as anger or loss of control are affecting your pain, then you will have no reason to engage in any type of rehabilitative therapy.

Some of us use denial to try to preserve our self-esteem. We may think that admitting that anything other than a physical problem is increasing our pain will lead people to say that all our pain is "psychological" or "in our head." This is not the case. It is known that stress factors at home and on the job can have definite effects on many aspects of our lives—including pain.

## Coping Strategies for Overcoming Denial and Acceptance

Acceptance of your back pain is vital for improvement—in both your pain and your attitude. If you can accept your back pain and begin proper treatment and counseling, you can look forward to lessening both your pain and your stress. Try these suggestions:

1. Keep a daily log of your actions and feelings and the intensity of your pain. Ask a counselor or someone trained in pain management to analyze the log and give you helpful suggestions for lessening the pain and feelings of denial.

2. Work on accepting the level of pain that you are experiencing, and focus your efforts on managing your life with the existing pain. Any decrease in pain can then be an unexpected surprise rather than an expected occurrence.
3. Do not equate seeking psychological assistance in dealing with pain with the assumption that people think your pain is in your head.
4. Accept the possibility that you could benefit by stress management techniques.
5. Keep an open mind to nonmedical alternatives such as biofeedback, relaxation, and counseling.

## Depression

If you have not experienced some degree of depression with your chronic back pain, then your situation is unusual. It is common for individuals in pain to encounter some degree of depression. The intensity and frequency can vary from momentary sadness to complete immobilization and suicidal thoughts.

You may consider yourself very strong and not subject to emotional reactions such as depression. Remember, though, that depressive symptoms can include mood swings, loss of interest in activities such as hobbies and going out of the house, avoidance of special friends, excessive sleep or lack of sleep, reduced or increased appetite, and difficulty concentrating.

On the other hand, you may be well aware that you are depressed. Uncontrollable tearfulness, feelings of helplessness or hopelessness, loss of self-worth, and suicidal thoughts or plans may have all come in turn. If they have, you must contact a professional—do not resist getting help as soon as possible!

## Coping Strategies for Combating Depression

Depression can be very serious and may need specialized medical treatment. For mild or temporary depression, however, you can begin today to understand your thoughts and emotions and move forward with a better attitude for living.

1. Never keep suicidal thoughts to yourself. Let someone help you.

2. See a qualified mental health specialist if depression is immobilizing you.
3. Never use alcohol or nonprescribed drugs to combat depression.
4. Seek counseling to explore the relationship between depression and pain. It can be very confusing to you and others.
5. Exercise is a great cure for depression. With your physician, determine what you can do to become active.
6. Never stay in bed all day unless advised to do so by your doctor.

## Anxiety and Fears

People with chronic back pain have legitimate fears of the future: How much worse will I get? Will I be able to keep my job? Can I continue to care for my children? Will I be an invalid?

Instead of being obsessed with these issues, you need to acknowledge your fears and channel your energy into positive action to either stop the deteriorating process or slow the rate of change.

## Coping Strategies for Alleviating Anxiety and Fears

Anxiety can mimic all types of illnesses with symptoms of nervousness, tingling in the hands, shortness of breath, panic, and more. Carefully assess your anxiety level and seek help if you have unusual symptoms or fears. Start with these recommendations:

1. Identify anxiety-provoking situations and try to avoid them when possible.
2. Discuss your concerns with a professional—do not expect a family member to be your therapist.
3. Have an open mind about interventions that can help you relax, such as biofeedback.
4. Join a support group of back pain patients.

5. Ask your doctor to explain to your family why you do better on some days than on others.

## Loss of Self-Esteem

Chronic back pain can lead to loss of job, decreased contact with friends, and reduction in leisure activities. For many of us, our entire self-esteem is wrapped up in one or all of these aspects. Now, when someone says "What do you do?", you may not respond with "I'm a clerk" or "I'm a manager." Instead, you think to yourself, "I'm a failure" or "I sit home all day." When you no longer have an occupation with which to identify, your self-worth may suffer.

One 50-year-old man told us he felt like a "bum" because his career in banking had ended so abruptly. "I feel like I have no purpose in life now," he said. "I get up each morning and sit around all day."

Being with friends and doing things for them and your family may have been your identity. Instead of being able to take an entire meal over to a sick friend or driving your neighbor to have his car fixed, you are now the one who needs help. If you have been a very independent person, this switch to dependency has probably taken its toll on your self-confidence.

## Coping Strategies for Combating Low Self-Esteem

*You can determine* how you feel each day, if you make an effort to find something positive to believe in and to look forward to. When you begin to have depressing or negative thoughts, remind yourself of a special award or achievement you received in years past. Let these suggestions help you fight low self-esteem as you take control of your back pain:

1. Make a list of all your good qualities.
2. Take the focus off the negative aspect of your life.
3. Remember that your family loves you for more than the paycheck you brought home.

4. Allow yourself to consider less demanding or at-home jobs that would occupy your time and make you feel worthwhile.
5. Do not avoid social interactions. Isolating yourself will only make things worse.
6. Try to do as many things for yourself as you can. You will feel better, the more independent you become.

## Guilt

You are likely to have some degree of guilt about having time off from work and being dependent on others. Guilt generally centers around three major areas:

1. Money;
2. Pulling your own weight;
3. Infringing on other people's time for help.

If you were the major breadwinner and have not been working for an extended time, you may be feeling guilty about not providing for your family as you think you should. This type of guilt can also be felt by secondary breadwinners or simply because extensive medical bills are an additional financial burden.

Jobs within the home, for which you were once entirely responsible, may now be impossible to complete. This leaves you with a sense of shirking your responsibilities. Furthermore, it may frustrate you that no one else does them, and you may find yourself getting angry at others over unfinished jobs. When you realize that those duties were always yours, guilt may set in.

Finally, not only is it impossible to perform your usual duties, but sometimes family members must take time to help you with simple things that you could always do for yourself before. If you dislike that dependent feeling, you are bound to become riddled with guilt.

## Coping Strategies for Dealing with Guilt

Guilt is especially difficult for someone who has always been "in charge," either in the home or on the job. Remember, there are still some areas in which you are quite capable and which you can control. Attack your guilt with these measures:

1. Accept guilt as a normal human feeling over which you have minimal control.
2. Try your best to do as many things for yourself as you can.
3. Never ask someone else to do something you can do.
4. Do not live in the past—work on changing the future.

## Fatigue

After having back pain for months, you are very likely to be worn to a frazzle, both physically and mentally. You have days when you feel that it would be impossible to move another muscle, even if you had to. You are tired of trips to the doctor, not being able to go out with friends, constantly hurting with every move, and just plain tired of being tired!

As strange as this may sound, the cure for this type of fatigue is often exercise. Many people do not believe this because they are so accustomed to solving fatigue with rest. However, exercise—not rest—can build up your stamina.

## Coping Strategies for Fatigue

Fatigue is often a symptom of stress. Instead of going back to sleep each day, make yourself get up at a certain time and follow a regular schedule of exercise and healthful living.

1. Consult your doctor for an appropriate exercise program.
2. If your doctor agrees, participate in physical therapy with a therapist who is familiar with chronic pain.
3. Use relaxation techniques for insomnia. If you are unfamiliar with these, consult a counselor.
4. Because stress leads to fatigue, avoid stress or at least learn to manage it.
5. Anger and tension also lead to fatigue. Avoid situations that bring these types of feelings.
6. Exercise regularly as recommended by your physician—no exceptions, please!

## Manage Your Stress and Seek Help

There may be other issues facing you. Because of the added stress of chronic back pain, you may feel that everyday stresses affect you more than they used to.

Remember that you do not have to go through this alone. Never be afraid or ashamed to ask for help. Trained professionals are ready to guide you and your family in a positive direction.

CHAPTER NINE

# Travel with Back Pain

We often see people with back pain who worry that they can no longer be active and travel. Some cancel plans and become gradually more withdrawn because of the pain. Limiting activity and travel, however, can contribute to patients' feelings of loss of independence and loss of control over their lives. Travel is important as a way to maintain independence, increase your sense of well-being, and continue lifelong learning.

It is not necessary to stop activities, including travel, because of back pain. Obtain proper diagnosis and treatment of your back pain and ask for advice on the needed *exercises*. You can take this key part of the treatment of your back pain with you anywhere in the world.

## Planning Is Important

You can consider almost all domestic destinations and even some international travel. (Save the rock climbing in the Alps for another time.) In most cases, there should be few major limitations due to back pain alone, if you are careful about planning and preparation.

Take a few simple steps to make traveling with back pain much easier. Plan details before you leave. Ask a travel agent to help you arrange a trip to a destination that fits your needs. For example, do you want a relaxing time at the beach or mountains? Or a visit to a large city for sightseeing? If you are careful, you can match your destination to a level of activity that fits your needs at the time of a particular trip. At a later time, your needs may be changed, depending on how you improve.

Plan ahead with exercise. Be careful to maintain a good exercise program for several weeks before you travel. This preparation will ensure that your flexibility and strength are at a high level for the trip. Try to be as rested as possible on the day you leave.

## Don't Overpack

Pack lightly. Try not to be caught in an airport, hotel, or tour bus with several heavy pieces of luggage. Carrying heavy luggage can cause more pain and fatigue and ruin your entire trip. Remember that you may not always have help available to carry luggage. Arthur Frommer, the dean of American travel, suggests that you pack one or two small bags that you can carry on your shoulder.

One good rule of thumb is to look at the clothes you plan to take on the trip and then take only half of them. Usually, you will do very well even if it means washing out some pieces of clothing in your hotel room occasionally.

You will enjoy the freedom from heavy luggage more than you'll miss the extra clothes. It isn't necessary to take clothes for every possible occasion—you probably won't be invited to meet a queen or president. Try to limit your bags to no more than 10 to 25 pounds total weight. You will be glad you did.

## Travel at Nonpeak Hours

Your travel agent can arrange for you to travel at nonpeak hours. This will give you a better chance for help with your luggage and avoidance of more back pain. Ride in an electric cart to avoid long walks in airports if your back is more painful that day. The cart can be requested when you make your reservation or on the day of your flight, and it will be available at the terminal upon your arrival. If you travel at busier times, you may find it harder to get this help in an airport, so try to schedule your travel at other than peak times.

## Fly Nonstop Planes to Avoid Carrying Luggage

Try to arrange for nonstop flights whenever possible. This will mean less changing of planes, less carrying of luggage (if you're switching to another airline), less standing, and less walking. Nonstop travel will also mean less chance of your flight being delayed or canceled, and less risk of added fatigue and stress.

## Have a Supply of Your Medications

Before you leave for a trip, check with your doctor to be sure that you have a full supply of each of your medications. At your destination, you may have trouble finding the correct product or finding a store that sells the particular medication that you need.

## Ask for Help

When you board your flight, don't hesitate to ask someone to help you put your carry-on luggage in the overhead storage area. This will prevent the strain of lifting and will leave more open space for your feet and legs. You should not be unnecessarily cramped and sitting in an uncomfortable position during your flight.

## Exercise Frequently during Your Travel Time

Continue your exercise program while you travel. With more time usually available, many people find that exercise is easier away from home. Walking is a key part of the treatment of chronic back pain and can easily be done wherever you go.

During travel in an airplane, you may find that your back pain and stiffness become worse when you sit in one position for a long time. You can help control this by walking up and down the aisle of the plane for five to ten minutes each hour. If you are traveling by car, plan to stop every hour or two and get out just to stretch and walk around the car. This can help prevent stiffness and fatigue.

Remember that exercises help keep your back flexible and strengthen the muscles that support the back. You can do some of the exercises in Chapter 4 while sitting in your airplane seat or riding in a car, especially those for the arms, legs, and neck. These exercises are especially helpful on longer flights or car rides, to help prevent stiffness and pain. They can also help make you less tired when you arrive at your destination.

## Select Accommodations That Fit Your Needs

Try to choose a hotel that fits your needs. Many hotels now have heated swimming pools or whirlpools that you can use for exercises and moist heat. In this way, you can easily continue or even improve your exercise program while you travel. It may not always be as easy or convenient as at home, but it is necessary to remain as flexible and strong as you were when you started your trip.

As a result of the Americans with Disabilities Act (ADA), domestic hotels should now have ramps at entrances and other facilities to make walking and general access easier. You may want to choose a hotel that has some rooms available with grab bars in the bathroom, toilet, or other areas. Your travel agent can help you match your needs to the right hotel.

## Pace Yourself

While at your destination, try to plan your schedule so that you don't do everything in one day. Try to fit in an amount of sightseeing or business that is reasonable for the time available. If you will be with a tour group, try to determine whether the group understands the value of rest as well as sightseeing. If you become too tired, can you miss a small portion of a tour to rest and recover, and then rejoin the group without needing elaborate rendezvous arrangements? Periods of rest will add to your enjoyment of the activities you feel you can handle.

In other words, pace your schedule of activities so that you don't wear yourself out. If you include proper rest, you'll accomplish about the same amount of activity without suffering more back pain, stiffness, and fatigue.

## Protect Your Back

Try to avoid unnecessary stress and strain on your back by taking a few easy precautions. For example, in a bus, plane, or train, sit with your buttocks against the back of the firm seat. Hold your back straight, not stooped over. There is actually less pressure on the spine if you sit upright in this position rather than slumped. Less pressure on the back will translate to less back pain and stiffness and less fatigue.

Protect your back from extra stress and increased pain. Take lightweight luggage, pack light, and use proper lifting techniques when you move or start to carry your luggage. Hold the handle close to your body and bend your knees when you reach down for the luggage, keeping your back straight.

When you plan visits to museums or other sightseeing spots, try to avoid carrying heavy camera or video equipment, and limit your shopping to small, portable items. Your back will be less tired when the day is finished.

If walking is too tiring or painful, don't hesitate to rent a wheelchair or cart. You'll see all the sights and keep up with everyone else, but you'll be more rested and have less pain at the end of the day. The quality of your evening and your night's sleep will be better.

Try to think of other ways you can adjust or accommodate your travel plans. The idea is to (1) avoid stress and strain on your back and (2) conserve your energy to prevent fatigue. These steps can keep you active while traveling with back pain.

CHAPTER TEN

# Questions Frequently Asked

Each day we see people with back pain who have a multitude of questions about how to prevent the pain, how to treat the pain, how to diagnose their ailment, and more.

Communication with your physician is important if you want to win with back pain. After reading this book, you may want to list any unanswered questions before you visit your physician, so all your questions will be addressed. Once you understand the nature and causes of your back pain, the treatment or prevention becomes more effective.

Here are answers to some of the questions we are most frequently asked.

***Q:*** *My back pain comes a few times each year and is severe for several days. The pain eventually improves, but it causes me to miss work and has resulted in loss of income. My spells of back pain seem to be getting closer together. What can I do?*

Severe back pain that lasts a few days, or a week, and happens a few times a year is one of the most common patterns. Unfortunately, no specific cause is usually found. The attacks of pain may become more frequent and limiting, and they can be expensive when loss of income is added to medical costs.

The best treatment is a combination of (1) moist heat, such as a warm shower or whirlpool, twice daily, (2) exercises for the back, and (3) medication to control the pain. If an over-the-counter pain medication doesn't control the pain, your doctor can help with a prescription medication.

You can continue to work if you are able to endure the pain and still function in your job. Bed rest does not seem to make the back pain go away any faster. Our patients make every effort to keep to their usual schedule while protecting the back from extra stress and injury until the attack is over.

The best and most helpful longer-term plan is exercise. Special exercises to strengthen the back have proven to be the most effective way to make our patients' attacks of back pain become milder and less frequent.

If you find yourself easing off your exercise program when the pain is no longer a problem, try to remember what the pain was like; you suffered physically and from loss of income. The trouble of an exercise program to keep the back strong is well worth the improvement and freedom from pain.

*Q: I was diagnosed as having sciatica, after I suffered severe back pain that shot down my right leg. What is sciatica?*

Sciatica refers to pain from pressure on a sciatic nerve, which travels down the back of the leg from the buttock. Pressure on the nerve causes pain in the area that the nerve supplies. There may also be numbness and tingling or burning sensations. True sciatica—pressure on the sciatic nerve—is usually from a ruptured disc in the lower spine which (along with surrounding inflammation) then irritates the nerve. (See Figure 10.1.)

Over the years, many patients with back and leg pain have been diagnosed with sciatica, even though many do not have true sciatica, or pressure on the nerve itself. Many other conditions that can mimic true sciatica are actually caused by inflammation in the soft tissues of the back (such as the muscles) or bursitis.

Treatment includes rest, moist heat, exercises, and medications. (For more information and medications, see page 12.) If

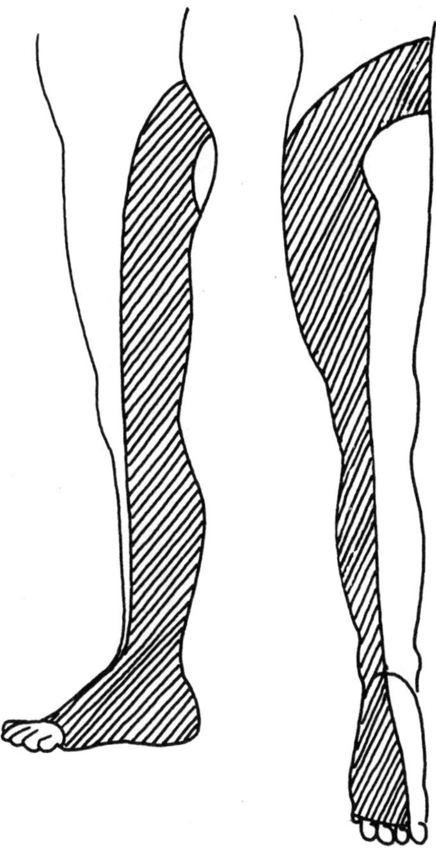

**Figure 10.1.** Sciatica may feel like "hot water running down the leg."

you do not improve, other tests may be needed to see whether a ruptured disc or other cause of true sciatica is present. Specific treatment can then be given as needed.

***Q:*** *I am 63 years old, and over the past year I have had pain in the lower back. It began gradually and mainly bothers me when I walk or do other prolonged activity. When I walk a few blocks, I have pain in the back that makes me stop. Sometimes the pain goes down both legs. But in a few minutes I can walk again. What can I do?*

You may have a problem with osteoarthritis, the most common type of arthritis, in the lower spine. The pain you feel when you walk and is relieved when you rest may be from pressure on the nerves in the lower spine. The way the pain behaves suggests the possibility of a problem called lumbar stenosis—a narrowing (usually due to changes brought on by arthritis) in the lower spine. This narrowing causes pressure on the nerves where they leave the spine. The pain is often most bothersome when the patient is walking, and it goes away if treated with rest.

The basic treatment for lumbar stenosis is moist heat and exercises. At times, relief results from one of the non-cortisone anti-inflammatory medications. Unfortunately, lumbar stenosis may not respond to this treatment. If the limitation becomes worse, surgery can give relief by removing the pressure on the nerves. If the distance you can walk before you feel pain becomes shorter and shorter, you should see your doctor.

Narrowing of the arteries in the legs, a less common problem, can cause similar feelings of pain in the legs when walking. This circulation problem is treated very differently, so it would be important to check with your doctor.

*Q: I am 49 years old and I worked as a welder for 29 years. I had several injuries to my back and haven't worked in two years. I have been fighting for disability payments because my pain is so severe that I cannot work. Now I have been told to see a psychologist! I am mad and frustrated. What can be done?*

Your situation is common among people with chronic back pain. One or more injuries results in chronic pain that make it hard to walk, bend, or perform their job activities.

First, be sure that you find any treatable causes of your back pain, as discussed in Chapter Two. Begin a basic treatment program of moist heat twice daily, exercises, and a simple walking program. Find the combination of medications that gives the best control of the pain.

If you don't begin to improve and increase your activity, other measures will be needed. Among them are nerve blocks, the use of TENS, and other treatments, as discussed in Chapter Three.

Often, it is very helpful to begin to deal with the stress caused by the pain. Don't feel that, because a psychiatrist or psychologist was suggested, your pain is "in your head."

Chronic pain causes stress, stress can cause very real physical problems, and these problems can make it harder to manage other everyday problems (see Chapter Eight for more helpful information). Psychological treatment can help you develop strong coping strategies to deal with the pain and your other problems. It is beneficial for almost all chronic back pain patients, not just those who acknowledge that they have "psychological problems."

Psychological evaluation looks at *you*—the whole person, not simply the painful back—and is an essential part of good and effective treatment of chronic back pain.

*Q: I have chronic back pain. Over the past few years, I have spent several thousand dollars on treatments and medicines that have not helped my pain. I still have to miss work. What should I do?*

Your story is familiar. There are many expensive ways to treat chronic back pain, but the best treatment is not always the most expensive. In chronic back pain, the best treatment may be the LEAST expensive.

First, see your doctor to make sure that no specific causes are present that can be treated and removed. Then, begin a basic daily (*every* day) treatment program: moist heat (such as a warm shower) and exercises twice daily, and gradually increasing amounts of walking.

A number of medications are available that can help control the pain. One of the non-cortisone anti-inflammatory drugs may help, especially if the pain is partly caused by a form of arthritis, such as osteoarthritis. One of a different group of medications (see page 51) can also help a great deal. Try to minimize muscle relaxants and narcotics. Pain medicines of other types are acceptable when necessary.

If there is no improvement over the next three to eight weeks, you should have an evaluation for chronic pain control. There are a number of possibilities for treatment of your individual pain problem, and some combination is likely to help.

In this organized way, you are most likely to find relief of your pain and incur the least expense. If a medication or treatment is giving no improvement, reevaluate it with your doctor. Is it necessary? Should it be changed? Avoid continuing treatments—especially expensive ones—that clearly are not helping.

An exercise program is one of the very few treatments for chronic back pain that should be continued in almost every case. It is the cornerstone for improvement and can be done at home at no additional expense. Remember that those who improve usually are those who are able to follow a regular exercise program. It does not have to be expensive.

***Q:*** *I am a 55-year-old woman, and my lower back hurts constantly. My mother has osteoporosis with a dowager's hump, and I'm afraid the same thing is happening to me. What should I be doing to prevent any problems, and do you think I could have a problem already?*

Osteoporosis is a common cause of back pain in women over 50. The amount of bone usually decreases after ages 30 to 40. If the bones become thin enough, then minor injuries or eventually only the weight of the body is enough to cause a bone in the spine to fracture, which can cause severe back pain. The fracture does heal, but it takes a few weeks. (See Figure 10.2.)

When the fracture heals, the pain improves or may even go away. If the problem of osteoporosis is discovered, good treatment now available can actually increase the amount of bone present, which may result in fewer fractures.

The goal of treatment in osteoporosis is to strengthen the bones and prevent the NEXT fracture. Hip fracture is the most dangerous. A hip fracture requires surgery, which carries its own risks. Up to twenty percent of older patients who suffer a broken hip die within a year.

If you have certain risk factors for osteoporosis, then you may already be affected, even without symptoms. Osteoporosis is not random—females who are over 40, white, and have had menopause are at higher risk. If you smoke cigarettes, do not have a regular exercise program, and have had low calcium intake for years, you are at higher risk. If other family members are affected, you are also at higher risk. The more risk factors

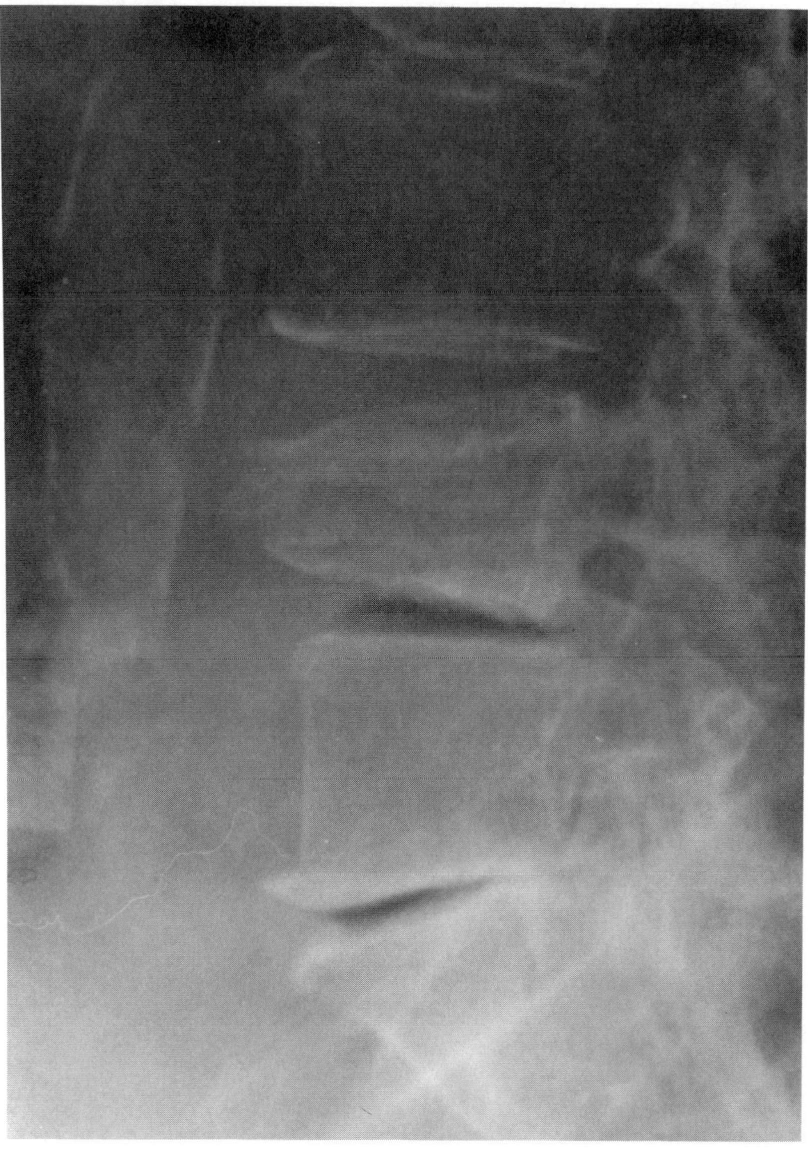

**Figure 10.2.** X-rays of a fractured spine.

you have, the more likely osteoporosis is present with the potential for fractures. By age 65, as many as 80 percent of women may have osteoporosis.

If you have more than two or three risk factors for osteoporosis, it may be a good idea to have a bone density test. This is a simple and safe way to tell whether you need treatment to prevent fractures.

The dowager's hump, the stooped posture that happens in many older women, is often caused by osteoporosis. The bones of the spine change shape: they become shorter and allow the back to become stooped. (See Figure 10.3.) This may be the only sign of osteoporosis until a major fracture occurs.

The best advice is check your risk factors. If you have more than two or three risk factors, begin specific prevention measures as outlined in Chapter Five. If a bone density test shows that osteoporosis is already present (remember that few symptoms will tell of osteoporosis before a fracture), start

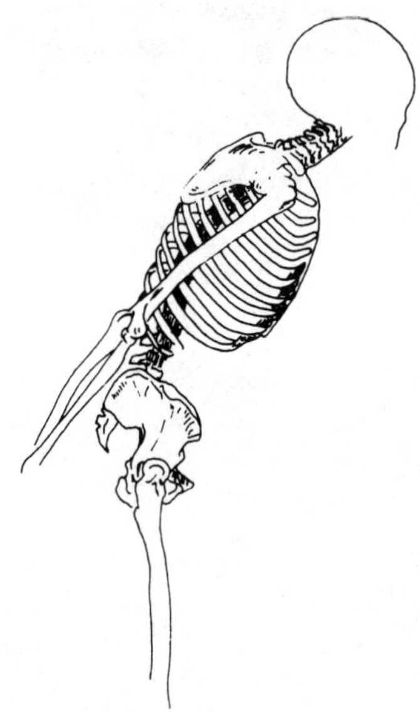

**Figure 10.3.** The dowager's hump. (Note that the lowest ribs almost touch the pelvis.

treatment to strengthen your bones. You may be able to avoid future fractures.

*Q: I am a 29-year-old man and I work for a parcel service, in its warehouse. I suffer from lower back pain from time to time. I need to work and I honestly enjoy my job, but I live in constant fear that I'm going to injure my back beyond repair and be unemployed. What should I be doing to ease my fears?*

You can help prevent back pain and loss of time from your job with a few simple steps. You should definitely begin an exercise program to strengthen your back muscles. You can start with a simple program at home, using the exercises for the back that begin on page 59.

Once you can do 20 repetitions of each of these exercises twice daily, you may want to add weights or resistance, using machines that can be found in a health club or gym. Swimming is another excellent exercise for the back. The more you maintain a regular exercise program, the better support you're giving your back.

In Chapter Five, you'll find ways to prevent unnecessary injury to the back from lifting. Learning to lift properly is easy and very important. Lifting alone accounts for many cases of back injury. If a load is too heavy for you to lift, get help or use mechanical assistance.

Back supports are worn routinely in many jobs to try to prevent back injury. These aids do not eliminate the need to lift correctly, but many workers find that the added support they give the back and abdomen muscles is helpful. Wear a support if your job requires frequent or heavy lifting. The support may help and it certainly won't hurt.

A number of the tips given in Chapter 5 can greatly help in the prevention of back injuries at your job. Protecting the back is the best protection against back pain. A large utility company found that when workers were taught measures to prevent back injury, their number of back injury claims went down. Less suffering, fewer lost workdays, and decreased medical bills were the reported results.

*Q: I was told that I needed an MRI test to determine the cause of my back pain. I am a 49-year-old woman and I don't understand the need to have this test. What is all this about? Is the test dangerous or painful?*

An MRI (magnetic resonance imaging) test is done most commonly to learn whether there is pressure on a nerve (from a ruptured disc) in the lower back that may be causing back pain. MRI is not done in every case of back pain; the test is expensive, and most of the time it is not needed.

MRI is indicated if the back pain is severe, doesn't improve over one or two weeks, travels down one or both legs, or is accompanied by warning signs such as change in bowel or bladder habits or weakness in the legs. The MRI test can detect a ruptured disc, infection, or cancer in the spine. The test is not perfect; it has been known to suggest a ruptured disc that is not present. But an MRI allows most patients to avoid the myelogram, which requires an injection of dye into the lower spinal canal.

Most patients with ruptured discs do NOT need surgery. In only 10 percent or fewer cases, the pain doesn't improve or the pressure on the nerve causes muscle weakness or other problems that can be best treated with surgery. In these necessary cases, the results from surgery are good.

The MRI test is not dangerous; there is no radiation concern. In fact, the results of an MRI test could help you avoid a CT scan, a myelogram, and other tests that have radiation exposure.

The fewer tests you need, the better the long-term effect for you.

Because everyone is different, you should talk with your doctor to decide which tests give you the best chance of finding the answer to your back pain but are also the safest and least expensive tests available.

*Q: I am a 35-year-old man. After lifting something at work, I felt a searing pain in my back and right leg. The doctor who examined me said I had a ruptured disc. He felt I might have to consider surgery. How did this happen? Are there any alternatives?*

You may well have a ruptured disc in the lumbar spine. This problem most commonly causes pain in the lower back that radiates to one leg, often bringing numbness or tingling. The good news is that, in many cases, ruptured discs don't need surgery.

Treatment consisting of rest, moist heat, gradually increasing activity, and exercises—along with medication—usually gives relief. If there is no improvement in a reasonable time, surgery can mean a return to normal activity and work much sooner.

Defining a "reasonable time" depends on how severe your pain is and how it limits your normal functioning. If your condition remains totally limiting, then surgery may be advisable in a matter of weeks. If there is gradual improvement, the decision may be made to "wait it out" in hopes of avoiding surgery. It may take a few months, but the improvement can happen and recovery may be as complete as with surgery.

It is thought that the cartilage material in a disc becomes worn or damaged. When the disc ruptures, its contents bulge backward and press on a nerve that travels down the leg. The pressure and the inflammation around the nerve cause pain, tingling, or numbness along the nerve's pathway down the leg.

When the pain lessens without surgery, it is because the inflammation around the nerve decreases. When surgery is needed, the ruptured disc can be removed, but it is not always necessary to remove the disc to gain reduction of the pain.

*Q: I am a 41-year-old man. I injured my back playing tennis several weeks ago. I stayed in bed for ten days. When I finally got up to go back to work, I felt weak and had no strength. My back hurt beyond repair. What did I do wrong?*

Your experience is common. For many years, rest in bed for weeks was recommended as the best treatment for acute back pain. Patients were often hospitalized, for complete bed rest, for days or weeks. But it has been found that this treatment does not seem to make the pain improve any faster, and the muscles that support the back become weaker. In fact, in only a few days, the muscles begin to *lose* strength, adding muscle weakness to the problem of back pain.

Research has shown that, when necessary, bedrest should be as short as possible. With the common type of acute back pain, we try to get most patients up every few hours for a few minutes, gradually decreasing their time in bed.

As soon as possible, it is important to increase activity and begin an exercise program. In this way, the muscles that support the back can become stronger and more flexible. Researchers have shown that this more active way of treating back pain actually makes the patient able to return to activity and work sooner than with bedrest.

*Q: I am a 25-year-old soccer coach for a local high school. I've had my share of aches, pains, and sports injuries, but over the past year my tolerance must be lessening. I've had back pain that happens in the morning upon awakening, then again at night after I get out of my chair to go to bed. My back seems so stiff when I stand after being sedentary. What can I do to improve this?*

Your back pain over the past year may be due to causes other than injury alone. One cause of back pain in men is arthritis in the spine, especially ankylosing spondylitis (see page 26). This type of arthritis begins gradually with pain and stiffness in the lower back. There is usually stiffness on arising in the morning and stiffness after sitting in one position. There is often fatigue as well.

Once the diagnosis of this form of arthritis is made, treatment can begin to control the pain, stiffness, and fatigue. Exercises are especially important because this kind of arthritis can cause stiffening of the spine over time. The pain can cause the spine to become stooped and less mobile.

With exercises, the spine can remain straight even if stiffness develops. This will allow you to continue your usual daily activities and work. One of the anti-inflammatory medications can help decrease the inflammation in the spine that causes the pain and stiffness.

This type of arthritis is commonly managed very well by those men who are affected. They are able to continue working, usually at the same job, and most often can continue to be active even in recreational activities. You should be able to continue your coaching.

*Q: I am only 30 years old and have been diagnosed with chronic back pain. Although I'm not a great athlete, I do exercise from time to time. What I don't understand is why a young person would have back pain when my parents, who are in their 50s, have perfectly healthy backs. Isn't back pain something older persons get?*

Back pain is called chronic back pain when the pain has lasted for three to six months or longer. Although many older people suffer with back pain, it can happen at any age. Most causes of back pain don't run in families, so you can't usually predict that you will have back pain only if your parents are affected.

See whether your doctor can find the cause of your back pain. Then you can make a plan for treatment and control of the pain. Remember, some causes of back pain may have particular treatments available to get the best relief. It's important to find these specific causes when possible. For example, some types of arthritis that are more common in young people cause back pain. Or, some types of back pain could be helped by surgery.

It's good that you exercise from time to time, but with chronic back pain, it is very important to exercise EVERY day, twice daily, never missing a day. In fact, for most patients we see, if we could recommend only ONE treatment, it would be exercise, not medicine. We spend much time explaining the importance of exercises, and our patients who win with back pain are convinced that exercise works.

For you, the back exercises should be gradually increased up to 20 repetitions of each exercise twice daily. Do them on good days and bad days. You will usually notice the effect of the exercises over a period of a few weeks to a few months. Don't give up before they have a chance to work. The exercises become easier to do after you can see that they relieve the pain.

Other steps that give relief for chronic back pain include moist heat, medications, and the measures discussed in Chapter Three.

**Q:** *I am a 44-year-old man. My physician gave me an anti-inflammatory drug for my back pain, but you talk about moist heat and exercise as being important as well. Isn't taking the medicine enough to give me some relief? I'm afraid that exercise or moving around might worsen the pain.*

That is a good question, because patients are commonly given medication without a recommended exercise program to strengthen the back muscles. Medications alone may give some temporary relief, but in most cases they aren't enough to give long-term relief.

It's natural to worry that moving around or exercising could make the pain worse. There may be some discomfort when exercises are first started. Try not to let this stop you. It may be necessary to start with only one performance of the first exercise, then two repetitions the next time; gradually, increase the repetitions until you can do 20 of the exercises. As the exercise continues, the work becomes easier. After a few weeks to a few months, you will find that the pain and stiffness decrease. The exercises become much easier to do.

Most patients we see begin to look forward to the very same exercises that were so difficult a few weeks earlier. You will probably reach a point at which you'll feel bad when you miss doing your regular exercises. You'll know then that you have made great progress.

**Q:** *I tripped going down the stairs at school and injured my back. My doctor claims that I should get better within two to three weeks. How can I heal that fast? Can you give some suggestions that will speed this healing? I am a 23-year-old woman who teaches first graders. I need to feel better . . . yesterday!*

For the most common type of back pain (see page 7), it is true that within two to three weeks there should be much improvement. It may seem that severe pain takes longer to disappear, but if no other more serious problem is present, you can improve your chances of pain relief and get back to work faster if you follow the basic treatment in Chapter Three. This includes moist heat, such as a warm shower, twice daily; exercises that are begun slowly and are gradually increased; and proper amounts of rest—not too much bedrest—with a gradual increase in activity. Medications to control pain or muscle spasm may help make you more comfortable until the rest of the program takes full effect.

Remember, the main goals are pain relief and getting back to activity and work. Follow this program and you'll put yourself in the best position to get the maximum improvement. Once you feel you can handle the tasks that your work with first graders requires, it is all right to return to work. Just be sure to avoid activities that might start the pain again, especially bending and lifting.

If you don't have improvement after one or two weeks, you should see your doctor. After six to eight weeks, the pain should be almost completely gone. Then you can continue the exercise program—your best prevention against the back pain's returning.

*Q: I had a friend who had cancer and suffered from back pain. I have had lower back pain for a few months and am worried about cancer.*

One possible cause of back pain is cancer, but you should know that even though it is always a concern, it is not the most common cause of typical back pain. In fact, it is so uncommon that we do not routinely x-ray every patient who has back pain. If the pain is very severe or if it does not respond to treatment as expected, then x-rays or other tests are needed.

An MRI test, a CT scan, or a bone scan can usually reveal cancer if it is the cause of back pain. If cancer is your main worry, you should tell your doctor so that you can be reassured or proper tests can be done to determine whether any cancer is present.

*Q: I had severe back and hip pain and was told that I had bursitis. I was given a shot in the painful area and had great relief. Will this pain come back?*

Some types of back and hip pain may be so severe that patients cannot walk. The pain may come on very suddenly, without any known injury. Bursitis around the hip can be one of these problems. It is most often related to the wear-and-tear changes. Although it causes terrible pain, it is not an ominous underlying cause of back pain.

The treatment of bursitis can include a local injection, which often gives very quick (and appreciated) relief. It is possible that the bursitis may return. An exercise program may help prevent further problems, although no perfect prevention is available.

*Q: I am a 34-year-old mother of three boys, and honestly have no time to exercise. Lately, I have noticed that my lower back has a nagging pain, especially in the evening. Can I do anything to strengthen my back besides exercise?*

Yours is a common problem. If your back pain is from the most common cause, as discussed on page 7, then the basic treatment program would be important. Exercises are key to increasing your chance for *long-term control* of your back pain. Because you *are* a busy mother, shouldn't you try to find some time for exercise?

The ideal program would be back exercises done twice daily, working up to 20 repetitions of each exercise twice daily. There may be days when this simply can't be done. If you have to miss an occasional day, it is not a major problem.

If you can't find two times each day to exercise, try doing all the exercises at one session—40 repetitions once daily. Many patients find this more convenient. Or, if you have access to a pool, swim for 20 to 30 minutes each day. You may need to go to a gym or health club to create time for exercise; access to equipment and machines may make it easier and more fun. Another option is to exercise in a group session or with a partner.

Our patients often wonder whether their normal activity can replace exercise, especially when they are very busy during the day. Unfortunately, activity and exercise are not the same, especially for the back. You must find a way to insert exercise into your day. Once the back pain is no longer troublesome, you may be able to do very well with exercising only a few days a week.

Although each group of exercises may take a certain block of time each day at first, most people find that they are soon able to complete their entire sequence of exercises in the same block of time. Compare the time you invest in exercise to the pain, loss of work, and curtailed activity that back pain can cause. You will be of more help to your family if you can avoid back pain by taking care of your back.

*Q: I am a 49-year-old teacher. I fractured my back while roller skating with my students. It has been almost four months since the accident, and I am having a difficult time healing. I am still in a great deal of pain. Is it possible that I have osteoporosis, and what tests would be done to diagnosis my problem?*

If you fell when you injured the back, the fall alone may have been severe enough to cause a fracture. However, since you are a 49-year-old woman, there would also be some concern about the possibility of osteoporosis (thinning of the bones). There are no signs or feelings of osteoporosis until a fracture occurs. If you have osteoporosis, then this fracture may be a clue that you should begin treatment that might prevent future fractures, especially a hip fracture.

Check the list of risk factors for osteoporosis, on page 174. You are over 40, female, and have had a fracture. It may be a good idea to have a bone density test, which is a safe and accurate way to tell whether osteoporosis is present. If you are affected, start now to prevent future fractures.

*Q: I am a 52-year-old attorney with chronic back pain. My internist gave me one prescription: lose weight! I need to lose around 50 pounds, but how do I start? Should I do anything else for treatment?*

In most cases of chronic back pain, control of weight can be helpful. It would be important to know whether other specific causes of the pain are present that can be treated and removed. Your extra 50 pounds can certainly be increasing the stress on your back.

Weight loss, especially loss of 50 pounds, can be intimidating. Try to have a goal of loss of 1/2 to one pound per week using the new Food Guide Pyramid created by the U.S. Departments of Agriculture and Health and Human Services. (See Figure 10.4.) The most painless way to lose weight is to choose a low-calorie diet that is livable—no less than 1,400 calories per day. Keep your calorie intake strictly controlled, and begin to use more calories by walking or another simple exercise. If you don't lose 1/2 to one pound per week, walk longer distances until you do. (See Chapter Six for more information on safe and easy weight loss.)

Slow weight loss is more likely to be longer lasting than a quick weight loss of 15 to 20 pounds in the first month. You would benefit from asking a dietician or your physician to

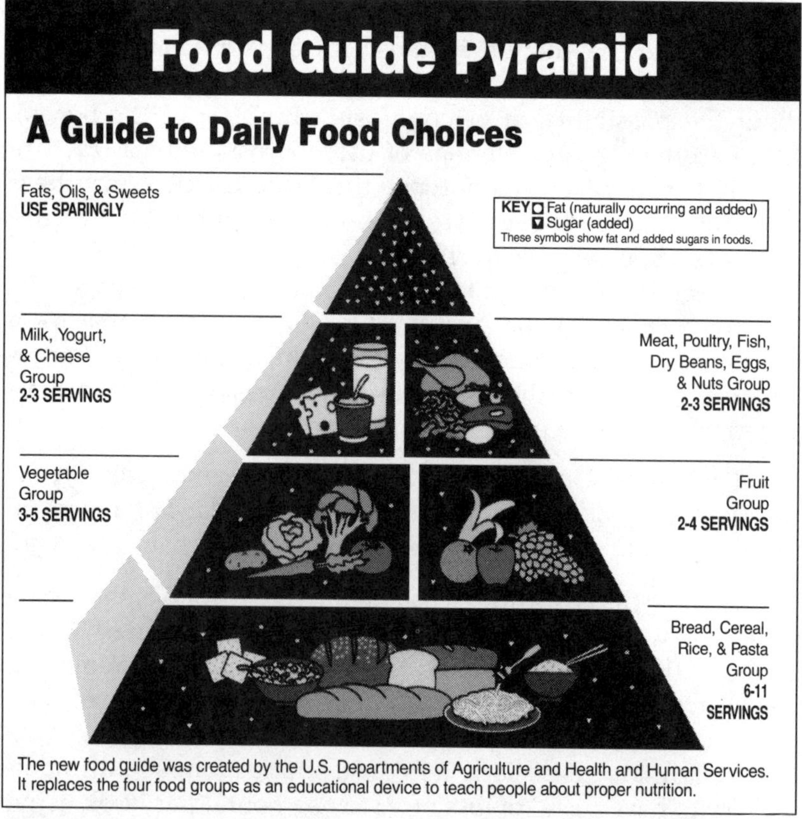


**Figure 10.4.** The Food Guide Pyramid: A guide to daily food choices.

help you make a safe and effective plan for losing this amount of weight.

Along with weight loss, exercises to increase the strength of the back would be important. Check your work situation to be sure that improper desk or work height is not putting excess stress on the back. Are you using chairs that don't give proper back support? Do your chairs fit the desk correctly? (See page 109.) The time you spend at a desk can increase back pain.

**Q:** *I am a 26-year-old journalist and work as a copywriter for a local publication. I have always had a strong back, but lately, when I get up out of my chair, my back is very sore and stiff. What am I doing wrong?*

It is possible that at least part of your back pain may be caused by excessive stress and strain on the back while you are sitting at work. The position of sitting in a chair and leaning forward causes higher pressures on the lower spine than sitting straight or standing. Because of this, sitting at a computer terminal for long periods can result in back pain and stiffness.

Using moist heat (a warm shower works very well) and back exercises can relieve the soreness and stiffness. The exercises will make the back muscles more flexible and stronger, which will help prevent future pain and stiffness.

At work, it would help if you could stand up and stretch or walk for a few minutes about every hour. If this is not possible, try stretching while sitting.

Try to use a chair that is comfortable, with arms that can fit under the desktop or counter, a firm back support, and proper height—your feet should be comfortably flat on the floor. Adjusting the height of your work to a comfortable level that does not require you to lean forward can help avoid fatigue.

**Q:** *I am a 72-year-old grandmother with arthritis in my back. I take a non-cortisone anti-inflammatory drug each day, but my friend said she only uses ice for treatment. Should I be doing this as well?*

Remember that there are over 100 types of arthritis. You probably are mainly affected by osteoarthritis (see page 26). In this most common type of arthritis, the cartilage wears or becomes less effective in cushioning the joints.

Ice can be used for back pain. Although most people feel better after applying moist heat, such as a warm shower, some feel more relief when they use an ice pack on the painful area for ten minutes or so. Some people get the best relief when they alternate moist heat with ice pack treatments. Ice may be especially helpful during severe attacks of pain. Choose the method that works best to give you the relief you need.

Also, don't forget the exercises that strengthen the back and make it more flexible. A walking program would be helpful—just pick a short distance and walk it daily. Then, gradually lengthen the distance as you can without increased pain. You'll be surprised at how quickly you can walk longer distances. Just be sure no other medical problems would limit your walking or exercise.

*Q: I am a 25-year-old woman. When I was in my late teens, I injured my back playing varsity volleyball. Although I have had no pain for several years, I am still apprehensive about the wrong kind of activity. My husband wants us to join a health club and use the weight machines. Would this be harmful for my back? How much is "too much"?*

It's important to know what type of injury to your back you had as a teenager. For example, the most common back injury among teenagers is strain of the muscles of the lower back. This can be very painful, but usually heals completely after weeks or months. You may have had a fracture of one of the bones in the spine, or any of a number of other injuries.

You may want to check with your doctor to find out what the injury was and to be sure that you can safely increase your exercise. Unless there is a specific reason preventing exercise, when you strengthen your back muscles you will HELP your back by making it stronger and more flexible. If you begin slowly and then gradually increase the amount of exercise, you are not likely to harm your back. Instead, you can make it stronger and less likely to be injured in the future.

There is no actual limit that makes exercise "too much," as long as you gradually increase. Begin with only a few repetitions and gradually increase the number; then slowly add light weights or resistance. Many of our patients enjoy going to a health club or gym. Exercising with others and with good equipment can be easier than exercising alone. The main idea is to achieve a regular program. You should do the exercises recommended in Chapter Four twice daily every day when you don't use the health club. Or, set your own routine of exercises at home. Do them after rising in the morning and before retiring at night.

*Q: I am a 21-year-old professional dancer with back pain. I try to stretch and exercise all day, but my back still has a sharp pain. Do you think I have an injury that needs further treatment?*

Back pain, especially chronic back pain, in a professional dancer should be given attention: the pain could limit or end your career. Talk with your doctor and be sure the back pain has no causes that need specific treatment.

Your activities may have resulted in a specific injury, and a short rest, without dancing, may be needed to be rid of the pain. Other activities can be substituted for dancing, to maintain your physical conditioning. For example, you may be able to swim or use other exercise during the time you are not dancing. In addition to strengthening the muscles of the back, this alternative would allow you to continue aerobic exercise and fitness with little stress on the back.

*Q: I am a 37-year-old woman. Is standing tall really that important? I seem to have great posture, yet I still have constant and nagging back pain. Even when I work hard at sitting properly at my desk and standing up straight, my back still hurts.*

Standing tall usually means trying to keep the back in proper position rather than letting it become stooped. When it becomes stooped, there is more pressure on the spine, which causes more fatigue, pain, and stiffness.

It's great that you maintain good posture, but that doesn't prevent other causes of back pain. In fact, the exact causes of the most common types of lower back pain are not known. If your back continues to hurt, you should try a combination of moist heat twice daily (a shower or hot bath) and the back exercises in

Chapter Four. Gradually work up to 20 repetitions of each exercise twice daily.

If your back pain doesn't improve after a few weeks, check with your doctor to be sure that no other problems are causing the back pain. It often takes a few weeks to a few months for the exercises to take effect.

There is no shortcut to building strong and flexible back muscles—exercises must be done regularly. But the rewards of improved control of the pain and less limitation are worth the effort. The longer you maintain the exercise program, the better the benefits are likely to be.

*Q: I am a 64-year-old man and have never had back pain before. Lately, I have noticed that when the weather changes, my lower back hurts. Could there be any correlation between the rain outside and my lower back pain? If so, what should I be doing to solve this?*

If your pain has been present over the past year, one likely cause may be osteoarthritis in the lower spine. This form of arthritis has been called the wear-and-tear arthritis. It usually comes on gradually, and many people notice worsening of their pain and stiffness at times of weather changes, particularly changes in the barometric pressure and humidity. The exact cause of this is not known, but the feeling is very familiar to many arthritis sufferers.

You can help yourself by following the basic treatment program, including moist heat twice daily, and exercises for the back. Over a period of a few weeks to a few months, you should notice an improvement in the back pain and stiffness. If you don't feel any improvement, see your doctor. Other problems may be present.

*Q: I am a 41-year-old housekeeper with a large cleaning business. I am constantly bending and picking up objects. While I have no problems now, I need to protect my future. What "back saving" plan would you suggest?*

It is difficult to predict whether you will have to deal with back pain in the future, but you are at risk because of your work as a housekeeper. Almost half of the adults in the United States suffer from back pain each year. The more frequently you lift heavy objects, the higher your risk of back pain.

If you carefully follow the plan for prevention given in Chapter Five—exercises to build strength, weight management, and learning the proper way to lift objects—you can avoid injury to the back.

*Q: I am a 49-year-old man, and arthritis seems to run in my family. For the past few weeks, I have noticed by back hurting upon arising, and I have wondered whether I might be getting this disease. How will my doctor tell whether my back pain is from arthritis, and what would the treatment entail?*

Your back pain has been present for only a few weeks, so the cause may or may not be arthritis. The pain may go away with simple treatment in a few more weeks. Remember that most cases of back pain are relieved in six to eight weeks. You can help yourself by using moist heat, such as warm showers, and beginning the exercises recommended for strengthening the back. (See page 31.)

If you don't see improvement in the next few weeks, see your doctor to be sure that no other causes of the back pain are present. Arthritis is a common cause of back pain; it is especially evident in pain and stiffness on arising in the morning or after a period of inactivity. Particular types of arthritis may be common among the members of some families.

X-rays, along with a discussion and examination, can help make the diagnosis about arthritis. The testing does not have to be extensive if no other problems are present. Treatment, in addition to moist heat and exercises, may include one of the noncortisone anti-inflammatory drugs for control of the pain and stiffness.

*Q: I suffer from chronic back pain. Many people don't understand how painful and discouraging it can be. How can I talk to other persons with back pain who can understand how it feels?*

You should consider joining or starting a support group for chronic back pain. These are small groups of people who form a voluntary membership. Members benefit by giving and receiving help to and from others who have a similar problem. Those who have chronic back pain can often teach others how to manage certain problems. They can help to fill the gap between professional care and family support.

A support group can help reduce members' feelings of isolation. They share with others their common problem, and many people believe that only someone with the same problem can truly understand how they feel. Feelings are shared in a safe atmosphere of trust and support. Members can trade tips on managing symptoms and emotions, and the supportive community can help to create a hopeful and positive attitude.

Support groups are not meant to replace professional therapy, however. Those who would benefit from standard psychological or psychiatric treatment should be directed to resources that better fit their needs.

Support groups can be organized by people who have the same doctor or clinic. The group can continue as long as it remains useful to its members. Over months and years, the group may change to reflect the changing needs of its members.

***Q:*** *I have chronic back pain from injuries in an accident. It's hard to keep from getting discouraged. What can I do?*

A strong and positive mental attitude can be your most helpful resource. Make a commitment to follow your treatment program—moist heat, exercises, medications, and whatever else is needed to get relief. Keep up the program on good days as well as bad days. Simply having a positive attitude seems to increase the chances of a better response.

Try to emphasize activities that you CAN DO. Keep up a maximum number of your activities, especially those you enjoy, even though you have pain. If your back will hurt no matter what you do, it is better to be active doing things you enjoy.

***Q:*** *The bills for my back pain are mounting—physicians, x-rays, medications, and therapy. How do I know if my insurance company will pay for them? I haven't filed my claims yet because I don't know which company to contact.*

Medical treatment for back injuries takes time and can involve medication, physical therapy, and expensive testing.

Treatment is generally covered by insurance, but the amount of insurance available may vary, depending on where and how your injury occurred. On-the-job injuries are generally covered by workers' compensation insurance. Injuries sustained in auto accidents are covered by a combination of auto no-fault insurance and group health insurance. Sports injuries and injuries incurred around the house are generally covered only by group health insurance.

Many physicians will file the necessary forms stating all services provided, but you may have to file your own claim to receive reimbursement. The process of medical claims can be confusing and stressful. If your claim is not processed properly, your benefits may be denied and your treatment may suffer.

Be sure you have all the forms you need when you file your claim, and take the time needed to fill in the blanks and to answer all questions. Medical claims can be held up or declared nonpayable when claimants don't follow the instructions. If a physician's letter must accompany the form, be sure to follow through with your doctor. Call your insurer after a period of several weeks, if there are doubts about whether your injury is covered. Most insurance companies have a patients' advocate available for detailed assistance on a claim.

*Q: If I strain my back at work, should I report it to my supervisor and seek medical care?*

Many back injuries occur while people are working. An on-the-job injury may seem minor but may prove to be serious if not treated. If you do not tell your supervisor you have been injured, you may have a difficult time proving that the injury occurred while you were at work. You should ask that a Notice of Injury form be completed to document the injury for workers' compensation purposes. The form will state the way the injury occurred and will describe the nature of the injury. If your employer refuses to fill out the form, you should report the injury to workers' compensation officials and seek the advice of an attorney who specializes in workers' compensation claims. You should also seek medical care to make sure the injury is properly recorded, diagnosed, and treated.

***Q:*** *If I am involved in an auto accident and experience back pain several days later, should I send my medical bills to my auto insurance carrier or to my health care insurance group?*

You should report to your auto insurance agent any auto accident in which you are involved, even if the accident was not your fault. You should also request claim forms or do whatever is required to put your health care insurer on notice of any accident in which you are involved. If you belong to an HMO, you need to schedule an appointment with your primary care physician. Most no-fault auto insurance laws require your auto insurance carrier to pay your accident-related medical bills and wage loss, whether or not you were at fault in the accident. If you do not report the accident, your no-fault insurer may deny coverage or your medical expenses and wage loss. Usually, no-fault insurance does not pay 100 percent of your losses. Group health insurance usually will pay all, or a portion, of the medical expenses not covered by auto no-fault insurance. If your auto no-fault insurance gets used up, your group health insurance would begin to pay your medical bills.

Generally, auto insurance pays the larger amount and group health insurance pays the balance. If you anticipate having a large wage loss, reserve your no-fault insurance to pay your wage loss and submit your medical bills to your group health insurer.

The relationship among auto no-fault insurance, group health insurance, and HMOs is complex and often can seem inexplicable. Seek legal advice soon after an accident, to make sure that your bills are being properly handled by your various insurers.

***Q:*** *Should I request a second opinion if my back injury does not respond to my doctor's treatment after a reasonable time?*

Yes. After a period of six to eight weeks, you should discuss your failure to progress with your treating doctor and explore alternatives to the current treatment program. It is very important to communicate to your doctor your failure to progress, and not just assume that your doctor has noted it. Most doctors welcome a second opinion in difficult cases and will suggest the names of other doctors who might be able to help. Be clear on your insurance company's policy regarding second opinions. (Some companies require them in certain circumstances.) This information is very important if your bills are being paid under workers' compensation laws or if you are a member of a restrictive type of group health/HMO system.

*Q: What should I do if my insurance company refuses to pay for either extended physical therapy or the purchase of therapy equipment that I can use to exercise at home?*

Insurance plans are intended to be general rather than specific. Your treatment plan may be outside the norm, resulting in a denial of benefits. If this happens, consult your plan booklet and find out how to appeal a denial of benefits. Be sure to follow all the procedural steps in a timely manner. You should ask your doctor to state in a letter to the person or committee handling your appeal why the therapy or equipment is needed. If you are required to attend a hearing, present all the reasons for continued treatment or for the purchase of equipment. If your appeal is denied, you may want to seek the advice of an attorney.

*Q: If the insurance company that is paying my medical bills or wage loss schedules me for a physical examination by a doctor of its choice, do I have to attend?*

Yes. All insurance policies that provide coverage for the payment of medical bills or wage loss have provisions for "independent medical examinations." The stated reason for such examinations is to verify that your treatment is reasonable and necessary, or to make sure you are still unable to go back to work. However, many independent medical examinations are requested by insurance companies to establish a legal basis to suspend policyholders' benefits. The suspension is based on the examining doctor's opinion that the treatment you are receiving is not reasonable or necessary, and that you no longer need to be out-of-work. Because the examining doctor is paid by the insurance company, a bias in the insurance company's favor could be present. You should advise your treating doctor of the examination and request that copies of your records and test results be sent to the examining doctor before the day of the exam, to allow the examining doctor an opportunity to review your records before coming to a conclusion regarding your case. You might also want to see your treating doctor earlier on the day of the exam, to have a record of how you were doing before the exam. You'll be required to gather up all of your x-rays and scan printouts and take them with you to the exam.

If your benefits are suspended as a result of the exam, you should immediately seek the advice of an attorney. If you contest the suspension, you have a good chance of having the suspension reversed. You should keep your treating doctor advised of all the details respecting the suspension. The examining doctor may have lacked some information, and your treating doctor may be able to clear up the confusion. You must realize that any treatment received after the suspension of benefits must be paid for by you. If your attorney is subsequently successful in getting the suspension reversed, you will be reimbursed for the medical bills you paid.

*Q: If I seek the advice of an attorney, what should I expect to pay and how is the payment handled?*

State and federal laws generally provide for the recovery of an attorney's fee if a person is successful in a suit to get an insurance company to pay benefits that should have been paid voluntarily. Many attorneys are willing to handle such claims on a contingency/hourly rate basis. In other words, you would agree to pay an hourly rate, but only if the case is successful. In that event, the insurance company would pay your attorney the hourly rate fee. If your case is not successful, then you would pay nothing except for the out-of-pocket expenses incurred by your attorney in the handling of your case.

Your attorney will want to investigate your case very carefully before agreeing to such a fee agreement, because no fee would be earned if the case was unsuccessful. You would be responsible to fully disclose all the relevant facts concerning your injury as well as any prior injuries to the same part of your body. In most cases, you should be able to get an attorney to review your case at no charge or for a nominal consultation fee. You would need to bring to the consultation conference your insurance plan booklet and all correspondence related to your case. You would also need to provide your attorney with a copy of your medical records.

# Index